Active and Passive Movement Testing

Active and Passive Movement Testing

Cheryl M. Petersen, PT, MS
Assistant Professor
Department of Physical Therapy and Human Movement Sciences,
Northwestern University Medical School
Chicago, Illinois

Russell A. Foley, PT, MS
Director
Georgia Rehabilitation Center
Newnan, Georgia

McGraw-Hill
Medical Publishing Division

New York   Chicago   San Francisco   Lisbon   London
Madrid   Mexico City   Milan   New Delhi   San Juan
Seoul   Singapore   Sydney   Toronto

McGraw-Hill

A Division of The McGraw·Hill Companies

Active and Passive Movement Testing

1234567890 DOC/DOC 098765432

ISBN: 0-07-137033-1

This book was set in 10/12 Times by Compset, Inc.
The editors were Julie Scardiglia and Barbara Holton.
The production supervisor was Phil Galea.
The cover designer was Mary McKeon.
The index was prepared by Jerry Ralya.

R. R. Donnelley and Sons, Inc. was printer and binder.

This book is printed on acid-free paper.

Library of Congress Cataloging-in-Publication Data

Petersen, Cheryl M.
    Active and passive movement testing / authors, Cheryl M. Petersen, Russell A. Foley.
    p. ; cm.
    Includes bibliographical references and index.
    ISBN 0-07-137033-1
        1. Movement disorders—Diagnosis. 2. Physical therapy. 3. Joints—Range of motion. 4. Human mechanics. I. Foley, Russell A. II. Title.
        [DNLM: 1. Biomechanics. 2. Movement. WE 103 P484a 2002]
    RC376.5 .P48 2002
    616.7'075—dc21
                                                                    2001031560

TABLE OF CONTENTS

PREFACE

This book came about as a result of a number of years of teaching manual examination and treatment techniques to physical therapy students enrolled in the professional and postprofessional programs at Northwestern University Medical School, Chicago, Illinois. In 1984, Steven C. Janos, PT, MS, OCS, began refocusing the musculoskeletal portion of the curriculum to provide a more complete, comprehensive and problem-solving approach to examination and intervention of patients with musculoskeletal problems and to improve and standardize the technical aspects of the orthopedic examination. William Boissonnault, PT, DPT, MS, and Russell Foley, PT, MS, were also involved in the development and instruction of the program at that time. In 1987, Russell Foley, PT, MS, Steven Janos, PT, MS, OCS, and Cheryl Petersen, PT, MS, began work on the manual that preceded the present book. Robert Johnson, PT, MS, OCS also contributed to the original manual.

The majority of the techniques included in this book are either taken directly from well-known, respected authors in the field of orthopedic manual therapy and neurodynamic testing (Freddy Kaltenborn, James Cyriax, John Mennell, G.D. Maitland, Ola Grimsby, Stanley Paris, Alan Stoddard, and David Butler, to name a few), or are modifications of their techniques. Emphasis is placed on being very specific in patient positioning, hand placement, direction of movement, and body mechanics. For the experienced clinician, such attention to detail might seem overly prescriptive, but for novice clinicians and students, this method is beneficial. With experience, techniques can be modified.

The present book was prepared to provide the student and practicing physical therapist with clear and consistent techniques to examine active (physiologic) and passive (physiologic and accessory) movement techniques of the upper extremity, lower extremity, pelvis, spine, and temporomandibular joints, and of neurodynamic base tests. It is limited to basic passive examination and treatment intervention principles, so that it can be used in entry-level physical therapy curricula. Relevant intervention principles related to passive physiologic and accessory movement techniques and neurodynamic base tests are discussed.

We are grateful to all previous Northwestern University Physical Therapy (NUPT) students who have used the manual for their suggestions and support. We especially thank Corie Jakes and Dot Berg, NUPT class of 1992, and Daofen Chen, NUPT class of 1995, for their assistance in reviewing versions of the manual for errors. A thank you to Sally C. Edelsberg, previous Director of Programs in Physical Therapy at Northwestern University for her wisdom and experience in assisting publication of versions of the manual; to Steve Janos for his assistance for revisions/additions of techniques for the book, Larry Olver PT, MS, for assisting and modeling for revisions/additions to the book version of techniques, and to Russell A. Foley for his support and direction of the artistic portions of versions of the manual/book.

We would like to acknowledge our family and friends for their understanding and patience.

PRINCIPLES OF MOBILIZATION FOR EXAMINATION

This chapter discusses principles of mobilization for examination using physiologic and accessory motion testing.

BIOMECHANICS

Motion Segment

The motion segment is the focus of active and passive movement examination. In reference to the extremities, a motion segment comprises the specific synovial joint and its associated structures, the tibiofemoral joint (Figure 1-1). In the spine, a motion segment comprises the two vertebral bodies with their associated zygapophyseal joints and intervertebral disc and the intervening structures, that is, the L4-5 segment (Figure 1-2). Motion segment movement problems are classified as either hypomobility (movement restrictions) or hypermobility (excessive movement) dysfunction.

Physiologic/Accessory Motion

Physiologic motions are joint and soft tissue movements that can be produced actively or passively, whereas accessory motions are joint and soft tissue movements that can only be reproduced passively. Normal accessory movement may be necessary to allow normal pain free physiologic function.[1;2] When pathology is present, changes in quantity or quality of these movements may be present.[2] Not all areas of the body presently have specific documentation of these small, millimeters of accessory movement.[3-9]

Joint Surfaces

All synovial joint surfaces can be classified by two geometric forms, ovoid or sellar.[1;10 p 499] Ovoid surfaces are egg-shaped, either convex or concave in all directions (Figure 1-3A). Sellar surfaces are saddle-shaped, convex in one plane and concave in another plane, at right angles to the convex surface (Figure 1-3B).

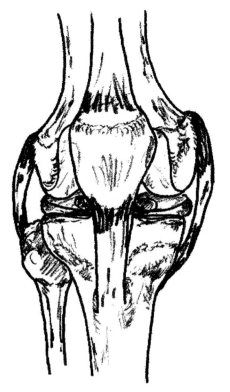

Figure 1-1. Tibiofemoral joint motion segment

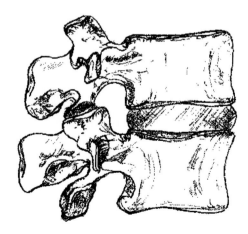

Figure 1-2. Spine motion segment

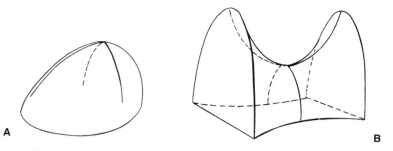

Figure 1-3. Synovial joint surface forms. (**A**) Ovoid; (**B**) Sellar

Six Degrees of Freedom

Physiologically, joints are classified according to the number of planes in which their segments move or the number of primary axes they possess; that is, the number of degrees of freedom. Mechanically, however, all joints have six degrees of freedom.[10 pp 498–499;11] Physiologically, the interphalangeal or humeroulnar/humeroradial joint functions with only one degree of freedom because of ligamentous/capsular and muscle constraints. But these joints[10 p 659] like all joints have six degrees of freedom mechanically: three angular (physiologic) motions in the sagittal (flexion/extension), frontal (abduction/adduction), and transverse (rotation) planes; and three linear (translational/accessory) motions in the sagittal (anterior/posterior glides), frontal (medial/lateral glides), and transverse (cephalic/caudal glides) planes.

Joint Play

Mennell's joint play describes the inherent slack found within a joint for normal physiologic motion.[12 pp 21–22] Inherent slack in a joint can be represented from two perspectives. First, it describes arthrokinematic motion, the study of the movement of the articular surfaces (accessory roll, spin, and glide movements) in relation to the direction of movement of the distal extremity of the bone (osteokinematics).[1] Second, it describes the passive examination of all physiologic motion end-feels (sensations perceived at the end of a passive movement) termed an overpressure.

Overpressures are performed by applying additional force after resistance to the physiologic motion tested is felt. With normal unrestricted motion, tissues, such as skin, fascia, fat, muscle, ligament, joint capsule, bursa, nerve, blood vessels, and joint surfaces, create the normal end-feel for that joint at the joint's anatomic barrier (Figure 1-4). When pathology is present, restricted motion may be found (Figure 1-5).[13 pp 32–35] Inflammation, muscle spasm, a loose body, tumor, fracture, scar, fibrosis, or calcification may change both the range of the anatomic

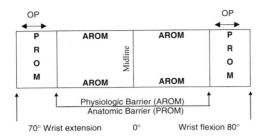

Figure 1-4. Normal movement diagram model showing the wrist's active range of motion (AROM) physiologic barrier and passive range of motion (PROM) anatomic barrier. Overpressures (OP) are performed at the anatomic limits of each physiologic motion.

barrier and the end-feel at the joint. Documentation of the quantity of physiologic motion is by goniometric measurements while accessory motions (roll, spin, and glide) can be documented on a 0 to 6 scale used by physical therapists (Table 1-1),[14] the 0 to 3 physician scale for hypermobility (Table 1-1),[15] or Maitland's grades I to V (Figure 1-6).[16] On the 0 to 6 scale, 3 represents normal mobility, while grades 0 to 2 represent degrees of hypomobility and 4 to 6 represent degrees of hypermobility. In comparison, on the physician's scale, which is used to evaluate sprains, 0 represents normal mobility and 3 indicates an increasing degree of laxity of ligamentous and/or capsular tissues. A comparison of the two scales can be made for hypermobility only, where physician's grades 1 through 3 suggest therapist grades 4 through 6 (Table 1-1). Using Maitland's grades I to V, grades I and II with an abnormal end-feel indicate hypomobility (Figure 1-7A) and grades III and IV indicate that the ends of range can be reached in a normal joint (Figure 1-7B) or indicate hypermobility (Figure 1-7C).

Overpressures can be used when examining passive physiologic motion. Each passive physiologic movement is examined at the motion's end range and information is found regarding the end-feel and the pain resistance sequence. Resistance indicates the end-feel produced. Pain that occurs before the end-feel is felt suggests an acute problem; resistance at the same time that pain is felt suggests a subacute problem; and pain that occurs after resistance is felt suggests a chronic problem.[17] An overpressure should only be performed if the passive motion is pain free. When pain is present during passive motion, an overpressure may aggravate the problem and should not be performed or performed with caution. To perform the technique,

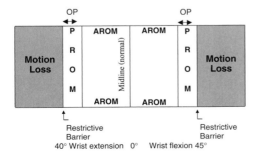

Figure 1-5. Pathologic movement diagram showing movement restrictions at the wrist.

TABLE 1–1. DOCUMENTATION OF THE QUANTITY OF ACCESSORY MOTION USING TWO DIFFERENT SCALES

PHYSICAL THERAPIST'S SCALE	PHYSICIAN'S SCALE FOR HYPERMOBILITY
0 = Ankylosed, no movement	
1 = Moderately hypomobile	
2 = Slightly hypomobile	
3 = Normal	0 = normal
4 = Slightly hypermobile	1+ = <5 mm difference comparing sides
5 = Moderately hypermobile	2+ = 5–10 mm difference comparing sides
6 = Grossly unstable	3+ = >10 mm difference comparing sides

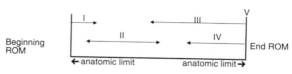

Figure 1-6. Maitland's grades of movement I to V for examination of accessory motion and for treatment intervention for both accessory and physiologic motions: Grade I = small amplitude movement performed at the beginning of the range; Grade II = large amplitude movement performed within the range but not reaching either end of the range; Grade III = large amplitude movement off the beginning of the range but performed up to the end of range; Grade IV = small amplitude movement performed at the end of range; and Grade V = high velocity, short amplitude thrust performed at the end of range.

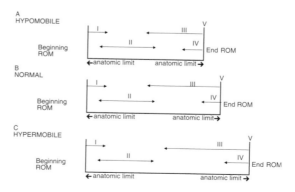

Figure 1-7. Comparison of Maitland's grades I to V for a (**A**) hypomobile accessory motion; (**B**) normal accessory motion; and (**C**) hypermobile accessory motion.

one joint partner, usually the proximal one, is stabilized, and the other joint partner, usually the distal segment, is moved to stress the ends of the physiologic motion examined (see Chapter 3). Documentation of each motion's end-feel (see Appendix 1 for normal end-feels), the sequence of pain and resistance and the quantity and quality of motion present should be included. There is some evidence[18] that abnormal pathologic end-feels (early capsular, spasm, springy block, and empty found at the knee and shoulder), present during physiologic motion, suggest dysfunction within the tissues surrounding that joint complex.

Close- and Loose-Packed Positions

The close-packed and loose-packed positions of any joint have clinical significance. The closed-packed position of the joint is the position where the joint surfaces are most congruent, where the ligaments are the most tight, and where the least amount of joint play is possible (Figure 1-8A).[1] Functionally, in the

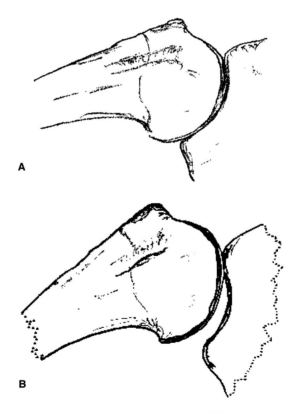

Figure 1-8. Joint positions. (**A**) Close-packed position; (**B**) loose-packed position

close-packed position, nearly all parts of the ligament are under tension so that a grade I/II ligament sprain should be painful. Because a large part of the articular surface is under compression in the close-packed position, an osteochondral fracture or degeneration of the articular cartilage should be painful.[19] A hypermobile joint may show greater accessory motion than a normal joint in the close-packed position. The loose-packed position of the joint is the position where the joint surfaces are the least congruent, where the ligaments are the least tight, and where the greatest amount of joint play is possible (Figure 1-8B).[1] Functionally, the loose-packed position allows the greatest amount of synovial fluid accumulation and therefore is the position that an inflamed joint assumes.[19]

PRINCIPLES OF ACCESSORY MOTION TESTING FOR EXAMINATION

The following principles must be considered when performing accessory motion examination testing.

Positioning

Consideration of the patient's position, maximizing patient comfort and relaxation, should be contemplated to minimize patient muscle tension. The therapist, as well, must be relaxed and use good body mechanics with close patient body contact to provide optimal control and precise mobilization.

Loose-Packed Position

Each joint is positioned in the joint's resting or loose-packed position (LPP) (see Appendix 2 for each joint's LPP) because the greatest amount of joint play is possible.[1,19]

Stabilization

One joint partner, usually the proximal or less-mobile one, is stabilized as close to the joint space as possible. Types of stabilization support include the therapist's body, the patient's body weight, a table, a wedge, or a sandbag.

Mobilization

One joint partner, usually the distal or smaller joint partner, is grasped as close to the joint space as possible to mobilize. Consider grasping a larger contact area to disperse the force.

Gravity Assistance

Mobilize with gravity assisting the motion or through the use of the therapist's body weight producing the movement, especially with any large joint complex.

Piccolo Distraction

Provide piccolo (considered a decompression of the joint surfaces) distraction (Kaltenborn's grade I traction)[14] before all gliding and rotation techniques. Increase the distraction force if any grinding or popping occurs.

Direction of Movement

The direction of movement for examination or intervention is related to the joint treatment plane (see Accessory Motion Definition later in this chapter)[14 p 13] and the concave/convex guidelines for each technique. The concave/convex guidelines of movement for synovial joints maintain congruency and contact of the joint surfaces due to the geometry of the articular surfaces. During physiologic motion, the roll and glide movements tend to occur simultaneously. Conjunct rotation, the automatic rotation that occurs with every physiologic movement, will always occur. The direction of the roll in the joint is always in the same direction as the physiologic bone movement, whether movement occurs in an open or closed kinematic chain. In the open chain, the distal segment terminates free in space (eg, the wrist complex during a hand wave) and in the closed chain, the distal segment is fixed (eg, the wrist complex performing a push-up). The direction of the gliding in the joint depends on whether a concave or a convex articular surface is moving. If a convex surface moves on a concave surface, the roll and glide occur in the opposite direction (Figure 1-9-A). If a concave surface moves on a convex surface (a plane joint), the roll and glide occur in the same direction (Figure 1-9B).[1,19]

Palpation

Whenever possible, palpate the joint line. Stabilization is more important than palpation when performing any technique.

Pain Free

During examination, techniques should be pain free. Do *not* push through muscle spasm.

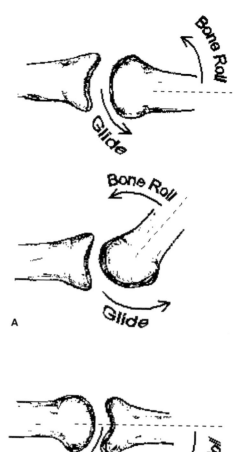

A

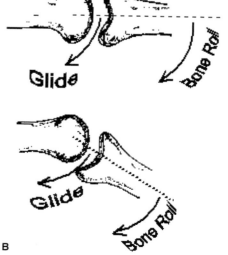

B

Figure 1-9. Joint accessory motion gliding when a (**A**) convex surface moves on a concave surface; and when a (**B**) concave surface moves on a convex surface.

Physiologic and Accessory Motion Correlation

Based on the concave/convex guidelines and the most normal anatomy within the extremity joints, physiologic and accessory motions correlate with one another (see Appendix 3 and under indication(s) for each accessory technique). Recent shoulder literature[20–23] does not support this concave/convex physiologic/accessory relationship. Movement was found to occur instead in the area of the glenohumeral joint capsule that was hypermobile or unstable and away from the tightened area of the glenohumeral joint capsule. This is a very important point to remember when intervention is considered. Interventions should be related to the examination findings and may not be specific to concave/convex guidelines for that joint.

Documentation

Documentation for passive movement should include the quantity, quality, end-feel, and pain-resistance sequence with explanations following.[17,19]

Quantity

Comparison from side to side for the extremity joints provides information about the quantity of accessory motion. Documentation for accessory motion, both for the extremities and the spine, involves using the 0 to 6 physical therapy scale,[14] the physician's 0 to 3 scale for hypermobility,[15 p 540] or Maitland's grades of movement, grades I to IV.[16] Quantity information for spinal joints is found by comparing adjacent segments within regions of the spine. Recent literature[5;6;24;25] demonstrates that there are significant differences in resistance between various spinal levels, suggesting that comparison between spinal levels is inappropriate.

In the thoracic spine, T5 was found to be significantly stiffer than T4.[24] In the lumbar spine, there is controversy over the relative stiffness of L4/5 and L5/S1.[5;25–27] Within the thoracolumbar spine, mean posterior-anterior (PA) stiffness was greatest at L4 and the least at L1; it then increased at the levels T10, T4, and, finally, T7.[28] Gender differences were not found to be a determining factor for spinal mobility.[5;19;27]

Spinal PA mobility stiffness is rate-dependent and increases significantly with a slower rate of loading. A therapist, therefore, should be able to push further into the range if the technique is applied slowly.[30–32]

There is instrumentation that measures spine PA mobility. Presently, two categories of instrumentation measure the force applied and the magnitude of joint displacement during PA testing. One type measures the physical therapist's performance of a PA pressure,[33;34] and the second type measures the force an instrument applies while performing a PA pressure on a human subject.[5;7;35-37] These devices may provide a means to train students and therapists to increase intra- and interrater reliability.

Quality/End-Feel

The quality of accessory motion should be described, and terms such as pop, click, crack, crepitus, catch, boggy, soggy, and the like can be used. Normal accessory end-feels should be capsular.

Pain/Resistance Sequence

The sequence of pain and resistance with accessory motion examination may suggest an acute, a subacute, or a chronic problem. Previous research on pain/resistance sequence suggests this information lacks intra- and interrater reliability.[38;39] Typically, the sequence of pain and resistance has guided intervention, but because of poor reliability, caution is suggested.[17]

Reliability

Research associated with accessory movement examination reliability shows the use of pain provocation is reliable, but the examination of the quantity of motion or the end-feel is unreliable.[40-44] New research suggests that the poor interrater reliability found when examining accessory movement end-feels and the quantity of accessory motion occurs because joint stiffness is a multidimensional concept.[45-49] "The question remains whether therapists have the sensory acuity to discriminate among all the characteristics of tissue and joint responses (mobility, resilience, resistance) simultaneously and, more importantly, along a continuum of such characteristics."[48 p 298] Nonbiologic stiffness stimuli (such as springs) are well discriminated even by inexperienced therapists/raters, further supporting the view that end-feels are multisensory and not mechanical phenomenon.[46;47;50] Further research is needed to define the multidimensional characteristics of joint stiffness and to develop protocols that will enable physical therapists to reliably examine accessory movements.[48]

Posterior-Anterior Mobilization

The relationships between the force used (greater than 200 N) and a larger contact area of the hand (the pisiform grip versus the thumb grip) are associated with a better ability to discriminate PA spinal stiffness.[49;51] The different strategies that are used when applying PA forces (an anterior force, a force applied normal

to the spinal curve, and a force directed toward the center of the vertebra) produce different loads on the vertebrae, and produce variation across vertebral levels.[52] The difference between using vision and the occlusion of vision during PA
mobilization has no effect on the ability to discriminate between stiffness stimuli. Under the visual occlusion condition, the same stimuli are judged as significantly stiffer.[53] The magnitude of lumbar PA stiffness is position dependent,
lowest in a neutral position, and increased in flexion greater than extension posturing.[54] PA stiffness is significantly increased with maximum activation of the
lumbar erector spinae muscles in normal subjects.[55] These research results suggest clinically important implications for the standardized use of force and angle
of force application, contact area, vision, patient muscle relaxation, and positioning during PA mobilization.

Biomechanics of Posterior-Anterior Mobilization

The force displacement curves for mobilization, specifically PA mobilization, re-
semble the force displacement curves of spinal connective tissues (Figure 1-10).
The segment below the level of mobilization receives most of the mechanical effects, both an anterior shear force and an extension moment (for example, during
a PA at L4, the L4/5 segment is the inferior segment). The specific level of PA
mobilization (L4) is subjected to a posterior shear force and the segments inferior
to an anterior shear force. The maximal extension bending moment occurs at the
point of PA mobilization. The intervertebral disc appears to be the major structure
that resists the anterior shear load and the extension moment produced by a PA
mobilization.[6;7] During the application of PA force to the lumbar spine, there is an
accompanying anterior rotation of the whole pelvis.[37] Preconditioning (increases

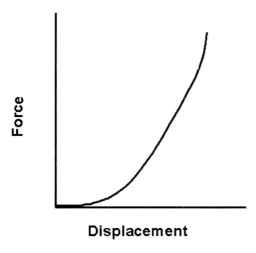

Figure 1-10. Force displacement
curve for a posterior-anterior
mobilization.

in PA displacements with cyclic loading) and creep deformation (increases in PA displacement when a PA force is applied in a sustained manner) might account for the improvement in PA mobility and active physiologic movement following PA mobilization. PA mobilization should be interpreted as a passive test of the whole lumbar spine into three-point bending.[6;7;37]

ACCESSORY MOTION DEFINITIONS

Joint Treatment Plane[14 p 13]

The joint treatment plane can be defined in two ways: (a) it is the plane parallel to the concave articular surface that passes through the joint; or (b) it is the plane lying perpendicular to a line running from the axis of rotation in the convex bone to the middle of the contacting concave articular surface (Figure 1-11).

Distraction, Compression, Glide, Rotation, Traction

Distraction, compression, glide, rotation, and traction are all types of accessory movements used for examination and intervention purposes. Each technique should be graded regarding the movement quantity (use 0 to 6, 0 to 3, or I to IV scales), quality (consider descriptors such as pop, click, crack, crepitus, boggy, hitch, catch, and the like), end-feel (such as Cyriax's capsular, bone-to bone, tissue approximation, spasm, springy block, and empty end-feels), and pain-resistance sequence.[17]

Distraction[14 p 24]

For examination purposes, distraction examines the mobility of the entire joint capsule and is the movement that occurs perpendicular to the joint treatment plane that increases or separates the corresponding joint space (Figure 1-12).

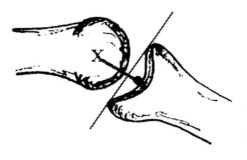

Figure 1-11. The joint treatment plane (line); X is the axis of rotation.

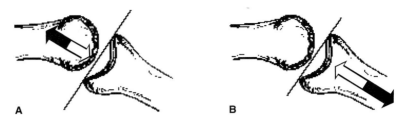

Figure 1-12. Distraction (black arrows) and compression (white arrows) for a (**A**) convex surface moving on a concave surface and for a (**B**) concave surface moving on a convex surface. The line indicates the joint treatment plane.

Compression[14 p 39]

Compression is most often used as a provocation examination technique in which a movement perpendicular to the joint treatment plane decreases or approximates the joint space (Figure 1-12). Pain reproduction may suggest involvement of weight-bearing structures such as articular cartilage, fibrocartilage, bone, the epiphyseal plate, or zygapophyseal/uncovertebral joints.

Glide[14 pp 19–22,26,28]

Glide is a translatory movement that occurs parallel to the joint treatment plane and occurs in anterior, posterior, medial, lateral, superior, or inferior directions depending on the joint (Figure 1-13). Regarding concave and convex surfaces, if a concave surface moves on a convex surface, the glide is in the same direction as the roll of the distal bone; when a convex surface moves on a concave surface, the glide is in the opposite direction of the roll of the distal bone.[1,19]

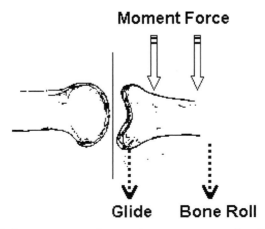

Moment Force

Glide   Bone Roll

Figure 1-13. Glide for a concave surface moving on a convex surface. The line indicates the joint treatment plane.

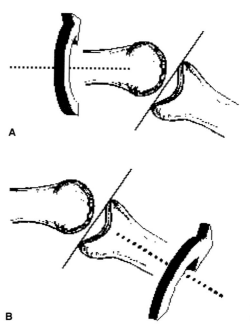

Figure 1-14. Rotation (arrows) for a (**A**) convex surface moving on a concave surface and for a (**B**) concave surface moving on a convex surface. The line indicates the joint treatment plane.

Rotation[14 p 17]

Rotation is a spinning motion through the longitudinal axis of the spinning bone (Figure 1-14). For every physiologic movement, there is a compulsory conjunct rotation that occurs due to the joint's contact areas, tightening of ligaments, and muscle contractions.[1:19]

Traction[14 p 24]

Traction is a separational movement along the longitudinal axis of the bone (Figure 1-15) that increases or separates the corresponding joint space.

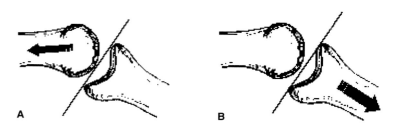

Figure 1-15. Traction (arrows) for a (**A**) convex surface moving on a concave surface and for a (**B**) concave surface moving on a convex surface. The line indicates the joint treatment plane.

INDICATIONS AND CONTRAINDICATIONS FOR JOINT MOBILIZATION

When using accessory motion techniques, the following indications and contraindications should be considered, regardless of which strategy — examination or intervention — is contemplated.

Indications for Joint Mobilization

1. To increase joint mobility
2. To decrease joint pain
3. To decrease muscle spasm
4. To replace a subluxation or dislocation
5. To reduce an internal derangement

Contraindications and Precautions for Joint Mobilization[2;56–59]

1. Articular derangements; that is, arthritides (acute problems, rheumatoid arthritis, acute ankylosing spondylitis); cervical spondylosis with vertebrobasilar ischemia; dislocation; hypermobility (Down syndrome, athetoid or ataxic cerebral palsy, generalized developmental delay); ruptured ligaments; acute whiplash; spondylolisthesis.
2. Bone weakening and destructive diseases; that is, fracture; malignancy (primary or secondary); osteoporosis; osteomyelitis; tuberculosis.
3. Circulatory disturbances; that is, aneurysm; anticoagulant therapy; atherosclerosis; vascular insufficiency of the vertebrobasilar area of the vertebral artery.
4. Disc herniation with serious neurologic involvement including compression of the spinal cord, cauda equina, and nerve roots.
5. Where infectious disease is present, examination or intervention of that diseased area is contraindicated. The infectious disease may spread with movement.
6. Pregnancy is a contraindication because of the alteration in ligament laxity and the potential for miscarriage.
7. Active growth plates in children and adolescents are vulnerable to linear and torsional shearing especially during growth spurts. Grades III to V may damage growth plates
8. Spasticity is a contraindication because of the potential difficulty in differentiating capsular tightness from movement restriction caused by spasticity. There is some evidence that the increased passive resistance that occurs with spasticity is a result of the presence of contracture rather than a result of reflex hyperexcitability.

REFERENCES

1. MacConaill MA, Basmajian JV: Muscles and Movements: A Basis for Human Kinesiology. Baltimore, Williams & Wilkins, 1969.
2. Paris SV: Mobilization of the spine. Physical Therapy 59(8):988–995, 1979.
3. Daniel DM, Malcolm LL, Losse G, et al: Instrumented measurement of anterior laxity of the knee. Journal of Bone & Joint Surgery 67A:720–726, 1985.
4. Hanten WP, Pace MC: Reliability of measuring anterior laxity of the knee joint using a knee ligament arthrometer. Physical Therapy 67:357–359, 1987.
5. Lee R, Evans J: Load-displacement-time characteristics of the spine under posteroanterior mobilization. Australian Journal of Physiotherapy 38:115–123, 1992.
6. Lee R, Evans J: Towards a better understanding of spinal posteroanterior mobilisation. Physiotherapy 80(2):68–73, 1994.
7. Lee R, Evans J: An in vivo study of the intervertebral movements produced by posterior anterior mobilisations. Clinical Biomechanics 12:400–408, 1997.
8. Pizzari T, Kolt GS, Remedios L: Measurement of anterior-to-posterior translation of the glenohumeral joint using the KT-1000. Journal of Orthopaedic & Sports Physical Therapy 29(10):602–608, 1999.
9. Sherman OH, Markoff KL, Ferkel RD: Measurements of anterior laxity in normal and anterior cruciate absent knees with two instrumented test devices. Clinical Orthopedics 215:156–161, 1987.
10. Warwick R, Williams PL, eds: Gray's Anatomy, 35th British ed. Philadelphia, WB Saunders, 1995.
11. Hibbeler RC: Engineering Mechanics: Statics and Dynamics. Chapters 20 and 21. New York, Macmillan Publishing, 1992.
12. Mennell JM: The Musculoskeletal System: Differential Diagnosis from Symptoms and Physical Signs. Gaithersburg, MD, Aspen Publishers, 1992.
13. Greenman PE: Principles of Manual Medicine. Baltimore, Williams & Wilkins, 1989.
14. Kaltenborn FM: Mobilization of the Extremity Joints: Examination and Basic Treatment Techniques. Oslo, Olaf Norlis Bokhandel, 1980.
15. Magee DJ: Orthopedic Physical Assessment, 3rd ed. Philadelphia, WB Saunders, 1997.
16. Maitland GD: Vertebral Manipulation, 5th ed. London, Butterworth, 1986.
17. Cyriax J: Textbook of Orthopaedic Medicine, 8th ed. London, Baillière Tindall, 1982.
18. Petersen CM, Hayes KW: Construct validity of Cyriax's selective tension examination: Association of end-feels with pain at the knee and shoulder. Journal of Orthopaedic & Sports Physical Therapy 30(9):512–527, 2000.
19. Evans P: Ligaments, joint surfaces, conjunct rotation and close-pack. Physiotherapy 74(3):105–114, 1988.
20. Harryman DT, Sidles JA, Clark JM, et al: Translation of the humeral head on the glenoid with passive glenohumeral motion. Journal of Bone & Joint Surgery 72A(9): 1334–1343, 1990.
21. Howell SM, Galinat BJ, Renzi AJ, et al: Normal and abnormal mechanics of the glenohumeral joint in the horizontal plane. Journal of Bone & Joint Surgery 70A(20): 227–232, 1988.

22. Poppen NK, Walker P: Normal and abnormal motion of the shoulder. Journal of Bone & Joint Surgery A 70:227–232, 1976.

23. Roubal PJ, Dobritt D, Placzek JD: Glenohumeral gliding manipulation following interscalene brachial plexus block in patients with adhesive capsulitis. Journal of Orthopaedic & Sports Physical Therapy 24(2):66–77, 1996.

24. Lee M, Latimer J, Maher C: Manipulation: Investigation of a proposed mechanism. Clinical Biomechanics 8:302–306, 1993.

25. Lee M, Liversidge K: Posteroanterior stiffness at three locations in the lumbar spine. Journal of Manipulative and Physiological Therapeutics 17:511–516, 1994.

26. Yamamoto I, Panajabi MM, Oxland TR, et al: The role of the iliolumbar ligament in the lumbosacral junction. Spine 15:1138–1141, 1990.

27. Nachemson AL, Schultz AB, Berkson MH: Mechanical properties of human lumbar spine motion segments. Influence of age, sex, disc level and degeneration. Spine 4:1–8, 1979.

28. Lee M, Grant GP, Crosbie J: Variations in posteroanterior stiffness in the thoracolumbar spine: Preliminary observations and proposed mechanisms. Physical Therapy 78(12):1277–1287, 1998.

29. Jull G, Bullock M: A motion profile of the lumbar spine in an ageing population assessed by manual examination. Physiotherapy Practice 3:70–81, 1987.

30. Daly CH: The biomechanical characteristics of skin. PhD Thesis. Glasgow, Scotland, University of Strathclyde, 1966.

31. Gilmore KC: Biomechanics of the lumbar motion segment. In: Gieve GP, ed: Modern Manual of the Vertebral Column. Edinburgh, Churchill Livingstone, 1986, pp. 103–111.

32. Bjornsdottir SV, Kumar S: Posteroanterior spinal mobilization: State of the art review and discussion. Disability and Rehabilitation 19(2):39–46, 1997.

33. Simmonds MJ, Kumar S, Lechelt E: Use of a spinal model to quantify the forces and motion that occur during therapist's tests of spinal motion. Physical Therapy 75:212–222, 1995.

34. Maher C, Latimer J, Adams R: An investigation of the reliability and validity of posteroanterior spinal stiffness judgments made using a reference-based protocol. Physical Therapy 78(8):829–837, 1998.

35. Latimer J, Goodsell MM, Lee M: Evaluation of a new device for measuring responses to posteroanterior forces in a patient population, Part 1: Reliability Testing. Physical Therapy 76(2):158–165, 1996.

36. Harms MC, Innes SM, Bader DL: Forces measured during spinal manipulative procedures in two age groups. Rheumatology 38:267–274, 1999.

37. Lee M, Svensson NL: Effect of loading frequency on response of the spine to lumbar posteroanterior forces. Journal of Manipulative and Physiological Therapeutics 16(7):439–446, 1993.

38. Fritz JM, Delitto A, Erhard RE, et al: An examination of the selective tissue tension scheme, with evidence for the concept of a capsular pattern of the knee. Physical Therapy 79(10):1046–1061, 1998.

39. Hayes KW, Petersen CM, Falconer J: An examination of Cyriax's passive motion tests with patients having osteoarthritis of the knee. Physical Therapy 74(8):697–709, 1994.

40. Maher C, Latimer J: Pain or resistance — The manual therapist's dilemma. Australian Physiotherapy 38(4):257–260, 1992.

41. Jull G, Bogduk N, Marsland A: The accuracy of manual diagnosis for cervical zygapophyseal joint pain syndromes. Medical Journal of Australia 148:233–236, 1988.
42. Keating JC, Bergmann TF, Jacobs GE: Interexaminer reliability of eight evaluative dimensions of lumbar segmental abnormality. Journal of Manipulative Physiological Therapeutics 13:463–470, 1990.
43. Gonnella C, Paris SV, Kutner M: Reliability in evaluating passive intervertebral motion. Physical Therapy 62:436–444, 1982.
44. Matyas TA, Bach TM: The reliability of selected techniques in clinical arthrometrics. Australian Journal of Physiotherapy 31:175–200, 1985.
45. Maher C: Perception of stiffness in manipulative physiotherapy. Physiotherapy Theory and Practice 11:35–44, 1995.
46. Maher C, Adams R: Is the clinical concept of spinal stiffness multidimensional? Physical Therapy 75:854–864, 1995.
47. Maher C, Adams R: A pyschophysical evaluation of manual stiffness discrimination. Australian Journal of Physiotherapy 41:161–167, 1995.
48. Maher CG, Simmonds M, Adams R: Therapist's conceptualization and characterization of the clinical concept of spinal stiffness. Physical Therapy 78(3):289–300, 1998.
49. Nicholson L, Maher C, Adams R: Hand contact area, force applied and early nonlinear stiffness (toe) in a manual stiffness discrimination task. Manual Therapy 3(4):212–219, 1998.
50. Nicholson L, Adams R, Maher C: The reliability of a discrimination measure for judgments of non-biological stiffness. Manual Therapy 2:150–156, 1997.
51. Maher C, Adams R: A comparison of pisiform and thumb grips in stiffness assessment. Physical Therapy 76(1):41–48, 1996.
52. Lee M: Mechanics of spinal joint manipulation in the thoracic and lumbar spine: A theoretical study of posteroanterior force techniques. Clinical Biomechanics 4(4): 249–251, 1989.
53. Maher CG: Stiffness judgments are affected by visual occlusion. Journal of Manipulative and Physiological Therapeutics 19(4):250–256, 1996.
54. Edmondston SJ, Allison GT, Gregg CD, et al: Effect of position on the posteroanterior stiffness of the lumbar spine. Manual Therapy 3(1):21–26, 1998.
55. Lee M, Mildren J, Herbert R: Effect of extensor muscle activation on the response to lumbar posteroanterior forces. Clinical Biomechanics 8:115–119, 1993.
56. Assendelft WJJ, Bouter LM, Knipschild PG: Complications of spinal manipulation: A comprehensive review of the literature. Journal of Family Practice 42(5):475–480, 1996.
57. Harris SR, Lundgren BD: Joint mobilization for children with central nervous system disorders: Indications and precautions. Physical Therapy 71(12):890–896, 1991.
58. Kleynhans AM: The prevention of complications from spinal manipulative therapy. In: Haldeman S, ed: Modern Developments in the Principles and Practice of Chiropractic. Appleton-Century Crofts, 1980.
59. O'Dwyer NJ, Ada L, Neilson PD: Spasticity and muscle contracture following stroke. Brain 119:1737–1749, 1996.

C H A P T E R   2

NEURODYNAMIC PRINCIPLES OF MOBILIZATION FOR EXAMINATION

NERVOUS SYSTEM FUNCTION

Examination of the neuromusculoskeletal system has historically focused on the various joint complexes. Recently, a series of techniques emphasizing movement mechanics of the nervous system was incorporated into the evaluation process.[1] Application of movement testing of the nervous system requires an understanding of the relationship of neural mechanics and neural physiology. These two factors constitute normal function of the nervous system. The relationship of neuromechanics to pathomechanics and neurophysiology to pathophysiology are continually being defined by the new pain science.

The overall function of the nervous system is to provide communication while adapting to movement. The first factor to be considered in the discussion of the normal function of the nervous system is communication; composed of two components, electrical and chemical mechanisms. Collectively, these components of communication are referred to as the physiology, or function, of the nervous system. These two components must be considered separately when determining pathophysiology through examination and using intervention techniques.

The most common form of communication researched and discussed in the literature is the electrical impulse, referring to the action potential. This includes sensory input and motor/efferent outflow.

The second component of communication is identified as a chemical process which involves axoplasmic transport. This chemical communication provides nutrition and receives information from the target tissue through axoplasmic flow. This flow is bidirectional and is identified by the terms *antegrade* and *retrograde transport*. These components of communication—electrical and chemical—must occur while adapting to movement.

Movement then, is the second factor to be considered in the discussion of the normal function of the nervous system.[2]

The connective tissue elements of the nerve are inherently related to the nerve's protection during movement while transmitting movement forces. This neural connective tissue forms the endoneurium, the perineurium, and the epineurium in the peripheral nervous system and the pia, arachnoid, and dura mater in the central nervous system. The endoneurium and perineurium provide the resistance to tensile forces, whereas the epineurium serves as a compressive force attenuator or cushion.[3] The new descriptive term that defines functional movement of the nervous system is *neuromechanics* or mechanics relating to neurodynamics.

As the body moves, connective tissues transmit forces through the nervous system while protecting the neural tissues from these forces. The neural elements undergo various mechanical changes, including gliding, elongation, cross-sectional dimensional changes, and angulations.[1;4] These mechanical changes relate to the mechanics of the neural elements.

NEURODYNAMICS

The normal function of the nervous system can be defined by the term *neurodynamics*. Neurodynamics is the relationship of normal physiology and normal mechanics (Figure 2-1).[4] The term *pathodynamics* identifies an abnormal component of physiology (pathophysiology), or an abnormal component of mechanics (pathomechanics), or a combination of the two.

An example of normal neurodynamics is seen when a high-caliber athlete is observed: extremes of range of movement occur within the athlete's coordinated

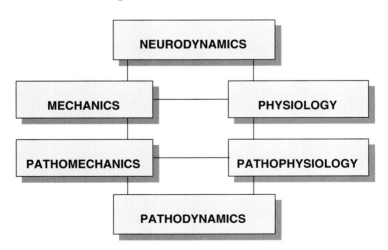

Figure 2-1. Neurodynamics comprises components of mechanics and physiology. Alterations of normal mechanics or physiology result in pathodynamics. Adapted from Shacklock.[4]

neural control system. The function of the nervous system, to provide communication while adapting to movement, is achieved.

EXAMINATION OF DYSFUNCTION IN THE NERVOUS SYSTEM

Review of Neurodynamic Tests

Evaluation of the neuromusculoskeletal system includes an appreciation of the interconnection between the physiology and mechanics of the neural elements. To test the physiology of the system, the conduction properties of the nervous system must be considered. There are a variety of established orthopedic and neurologic tests. The clinician may use any number of these tests including active and passive range of motion, resisted testing, sensory and motor examination of the central and peripheral nervous system, and electrodiagnostic testing.

Neurodynamic testing also addresses the physical capabilities of the nervous system through manual positioning and loading. This type of examination identifies the load characteristics of the neural elements. There are multiple techniques that use positioning and movement to focus tensile load through the neural elements or to unload the neural structures. These techniques identify the mechanics of the nerve or the nerve's ability to move, including the ability to slide, angulate, glide, strain, or compress. Additional responses are tension, changes in intraneural pressure, and alterations in cross-sectional diameter of the nerve. The nerve bed can increase in length from 12 to 20 percent during limb movements.[5;6] The nervous system has the ability to move, and this capacity to move has been described by many researchers whose work has focused on upper limb, lower limb, and spinal neural mobility.[2;7–9]

The load or mechanical force through the neural elements also challenges the health of the nervous system. Manual loading tests help to identify the physiologic reaction of the nerve to mechanical force. These physiologic responses may include alterations in impulse generation, changes in intraneural blood flow, or changes in axonal transport. It has been demonstrated that blood flow will slow at 6 to 8 percent load or strain of the nerve.[10] At 15 percent elongation, complete arrest of blood flow may occur.[11] Compression will also alter blood flow and axoplasmic transport.[12;13] Extraneural pressure of approximately 20 to 30 mm Hg will affect nerve function. These relationships are relevant to examination and intervention considerations.

Base Tests

There are many nervous system mechanical tests that are common to medical and physical therapy examination. These tests include passive neck flexion,[14;15] the slump test,[17;18] straight leg raise,[16] prone knee bend,[19] and upper limb tension tests,[1;20–22]

Butler[1] proposed a series of base tests to examine the integrity of the nervous system including both the central and peripheral components. These base tests include:

- Passive Neck Flexion (PNF)
- Straight Leg Raise (SLR)
- Slump Test
- Prone Knee Bend (PKB)
- Upper Limb Neurodynamic Tests (ULNT)

These tests are designed to bias (direct a force through) the neural elements to a greater degree than the surrounding interface. These tests attempt to load (direct force through) specific nerve roots, nerve trunks, localized regions of the central canal, or even components of the sympathetic nervous system,[23] but these tests are generally not that specific. The clinician should remember that mechanical loading will bias other neural and nonneural tissues as well. This neurodynamic examination information should be put into the clinical reasoning/problem solving framework to determine clinical relevancy.[24;25]

DETERMINING TEST RESULTS

Test Responses

Neurodynamic testing leads to a variety of patient responses. Some responses may be relevant to the patient's condition, whereas others may not be. It is important to put this information into the clinical reasoning/problem solving framework.[26] The patient's response to the tests may be placed into three general categories.

1. *Physiologic:* This is a normal response to neural and nonneural tissue loading. The sensation felt by the patient, as a stretch of tissues, is symptomatic. This might include sensations of deep or dull aching. For example, the responses for an ULNT, specific to the median nerve may present as a deep ache in the cubital fossa extending to the anterior and radial aspect of the forearm into the radial side of the hand.[22] Side bending of the cervical spine away from the side being tested increases this response in the upper extremity in 90 percent of normal patients. Side bending to the same side being tested may relieve the stretch sensation.

2. *Clinical Physiologic:* This category is when a response is elicited but the response is not the patient's exact presenting symptom or complaint. Compared to the normal side, the sensations created with the test are unusual. The test is not considered normal but it has not produced a clinically posi-

tive test response. This clinical physiologic response does not identify a specific area of local involvement or the specific complaint. The perception is that something is not right as compared to the opposite, normal side. This information is important especially in very subtle clinical presentations. The clinician now has a nonnormal finding to pursue to determine relevancy within the clinical presentation.

3. *Neurogenic:* This response defines the symptom(s) or a component of the symptom(s) to be originating from the nervous system. For example, a low back pain complaint that is not elicited with a seated, modified straight leg raise, but that is produced with dorsiflexion of the ankle maintaining the same test position, or the complaint is relieved when the ankle is returned to neutral maintaining the straight leg raise position. This is an example of structural differentiation, which is described next.

Structural Differentiation

Structural differentiation is a component of testing that assists the clinician in determining the potential involvement of the nervous system related to the symptom complaint. If the symptom is made worse or lessened by moving an area of the body or joint complex far removed from the local area of complaint,[27] it is said to be neurogenic positive. For example, during a SLR, the patient may complain of generalized hamstring or buttock pain. This pain may be increased or decreased with cervical flexion or extension. In this example, the common tissue and the only structure being altered at the buttock or knee is the nervous system. This is a neurogenic positive response. Because the nervous system is a continuum, it enables differential testing. Neural tissue contributes to the pain complaint in this situation and must be considered as part of the intervention plan (see Chapter 5).

INDICATIONS AND CONTRAINDICATIONS FOR MOBILIZATION OF THE NERVOUS SYSTEM

The nervous system can be mobilized like any joint complex, muscle, or fascia with similar indications and contraindications. The nervous system is constantly being mobilized with other examination techniques. A traditional hamstring stretch mobilizes components of the sciatic nerve. Any muscle stretching technique will mobilize nerve tissue. Neurodynamics is both an examination and intervention approach that attempts to bias specific or local neural tissue to a greater extent than other surrounding neural or nonneural tissue.

The indications and contraindications listed below should be considered when determining whether to use neurodynamic examination or intervention techniques.[26]

Indications for mobilization of the nervous system are:

1. To examine, normalize, or improve the normal neurodynamics of the nervous system. This refers to the understanding of the new pain sciences, including pathophysiology and pathomechanics of the nervous system, and to identifying nervous system pathodynamics with the ultimate goal of returning the system as close as possible to normal neurodynamics.
2. A clinical reasoning hypothesis of movement dysfunction supporting neurogenic pain.[24-26]
3. An aggravation of the pain pattern by a functional position or an activity of daily living position that resembles a base test position. For example, the position of the upper extremity during combing or drying the hair that is similar to the ulnar nerve upper limb neurodynamic test position, or getting into a car with pain provocation during neck flexion that is similar to the slump test position.
4. Positive conduction tests suggesting neural involvement.

Contraindications to mobilization of the nervous system are:[1;26]

1. Increasing neurologic signs or neurologic injury when a load is likely to cause a rapid neurologic deficit.
2. Red flags found with a neurologic examination, such as extrasegmental or multilevel loss of sensory or motor function, a positive Babinski response, or loss of bowel or bladder function.
3. Severe injury or abnormality of the interfacing tissue of the nervous system found with spinal instability, osteoporosis, transient quadriplegia, and the like.
4. Inflammatory, infectious, or viral conditions, such as an abscess, Guillian Barré syndrome, and the like.
5. A tethered spinal cord or conditions with spinal cord adherence to the meninges or the spinal canal.
6. Severe pain as a result of any examination technique. This situation requires extreme caution by the practicing clinician.

REFERENCES

1. Butler DS: Mobilisation of the Nervous System. Melbourne, Australia, Churchill Livingstone, 1991.
2. Millesi H: Gliding tissue of peripheral nerves: Its surgical significance. In: Hunter J, Schneider L, Mackin E, eds: Tendon and Nerve Surgery in the Hand. St. Louis, Mosby, 1997, pp. 111–120.

3. Sunderland S: Nerves and Nerve Injuries. Edinburgh, Scotland, Churchill Livingstone, 1978.
4. Shacklock M: Neurodynamics. Physiotherapy 81:9–16, 1995.
5. Beith I, Robins E, Richards P: An assessment of the adaptive mechanisms within and surrounding the peripheral nervous system during changes in nerve bed length resulting from underlying joint movement. In: Shacklock M, ed: Moving in on Pain. Chatswood, Australia, Butterworth-Heinemann, 1995, pp. 194–203.
6. Zoch G, Reishner R, Beer R, et al: Stress and strain in peripheral nerves. Neuro-Orthopedics 10:73–82, 1991.
7. Wilgis E, Murphy R: The significance of longitudinal excursion in peripheral nerves. Hand Clinics 2:761–786, 1986.
8. McLellan D, Swash M: Longitudinal sliding of the median nerve during movements of the upper limb. Journal of Neurology, Neurosurgery, and Psychiatry 39:566–570, 1976.
9. Louis R: Vertebroradicular and vertebromedullar dynamics. Anatomia Clinica 3:1–11, 1981.
10. Wall E, Massie J, Kwan M: Experimental stretch neuropathy. Journal of Bone and Joint Surgery 74B:126–129, 1992.
11. Ogata K, Naito M: Blood flow of peripheral nerve: Effects of dissection, stretching and compression. Journal of Hand Surgery 11B:10–14, 1986.
12. Rydevik B, Lundborg G, Bagge U: Effects of graded compression on intraneural blood flow: An in-vivo study on rabbit tibial nerve. Journal of Hand Surgery 6:3–12, 1981.
13. Rempel D, Dahlin L, Lundborg G: Pathophysiology of nerve compression syndromes: Response of peripheral nerves to loading. Journal of Bone and Joint Surgery 81A:1600–1610, 1999.
14. Reid J: Effects of flexion-extension movements of the head and spine upon the spinal cord and nerve roots. Journal of Neurology, Neurosurgery, and Psychiatry 23:214–221, 1960.
15. Adams C, Loque V: Studies in cervical spondylotic myelopathy: I. Movement of the cervical roots, dura and cord and their relation to the course of the extrathecal roots. Brain 94:557–568, 1971.
16. Brieg A, Troup J: Biomechanical considerations in the straight-leg raising test. Spine 4:242–250, 1979.
17. Cyriax J: Textbook of Orthopaedic Medicine, 8th ed. London, Baillière Tindall, 1982.
18. Maitland GD: Vertebral Manipulation, 5th ed. London, Butterworths, 1986.
19. O'Connell J: Sciatica and the mechanism of the production of the clinical syndrome in protrusions of the lumbar intervertebral discs. British Journal of Surgery 30:315–327, 1946.
20. Frykholm R: The mechanism of cervical radicular lesions resulting from friction or forceful traction. Acta Chirugica Scandinavica 102:93–98, 1951.
21. Elvey R: Brachial plexus tension tests and the pathoanatomical origin of arm pain. In: Idczak, R, ed: Aspects of Manipulative Therapy. Melbourne, Victoria, Lincoln Institute of Health Sciences, 1980, pp. 105–109.
22. Kenneally M, Rubenach H, Elvey R: The upper limb tension test: The SLR test of the arm. In: Grant R, ed: Clinics in Physical Therapy: The Cervical and Thoracic Spines. New York, Churchill Livingstone, 1988, pp. 167–194.

23. Butler DS, Slater H: Neural injury in the thoracic spine: A conceptual basis for manual therapy. In: Grant R, ed: Clinics in Physical Therapy: The Cervical and Thoracic Spines. New York, Churchill Livingstone, 1994, pp. 313–338.
24. Jones M: Clinical reasoning in manual therapy. Physical Therapy 72:875–884, 1992.
25. Foley R: Complex Regional Pain Syndromes: Focus on the Autonomic Nervous System. Adelaide, Australia, NOI Group Publications, 2000.
26. Butler DS: The Sensitive Nervous System. Adelaide, Australia, NOI Group Publications, 2000.

EXAMINATION TECHNIQUES

EXPLANATION OF FIGURE SYMBOLS

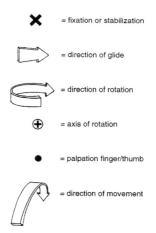

✖ = fixation or stabilization

⟹ = direction of glide

↻ = direction of rotation

⊕ = axis of rotation

● = palpation finger/thumb

↪ = direction of movement

SKELETON FIGURES

Some of the examination techniques will be demonstrated on a skeleton. This is done to more specifically show hand placement in relation to the joint line with removal of the soft tissues.

PRINCIPLES OF ACTIVE AND PASSIVE MOVEMENT TESTING/OVERPRESSURES FOR THE EXTREMITIES

Observe the patient in sitting or standing performing active extremity movements from an anterior, a posterior, and both lateral views prior to any passive movements and overpressures. Overpressures are examined when passive movements are symptom free. The quality and quantity of active and passive movements should be evaluated. Identify deviations from the normal planes of motion. When overpressures are performed, the end-feel and the sequence of pain and resistance should be examined.

UPPER EXTREMITY

Glenohumeral

Flexion Overpressure

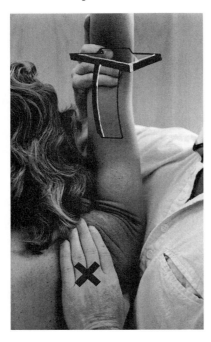

Patient Position: Patient sits or stands in neutral posture.

Therapist Position: Therapist stands alongside the patient facing the patient's upper extremity.

Stabilization: Therapist stabilizes the scapula in an inferior and medial direction (palm over vertebral scapular border).

Mobilization: Therapist grasps the patient's forearm either with the patient's elbow flexed or extended.

Direction of Force: Therapist's mobilizing hand flexes the shoulder to the end of range.

Glenohumeral

Extension Overpressure

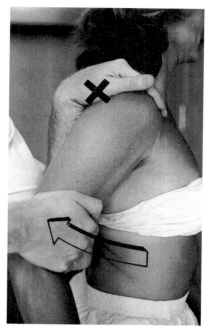

Patient Position: Patient sits or stands in neutral posture.

Therapist Position: Therapist stands behind the patient.

Stabilization: Therapist's medial hand stabilizes the scapula in an inferior direction (fingers over the coracoid process area and palm/forearm over the scapula).

Mobilization: Therapist's lateral hand grasps the patient's upper arm (patient's elbow relaxed in slight flexion or extension).

Direction of Force: Therapist's mobilizing hand extends the shoulder to the end of range.

Glenohumeral

Abduction Overpressure Positioning

To accurately assess pure passive glenohumeral abduction with an overpressure, it is important to specifically position the patient's upper extremity in the plane of the scapula (this allows for patient-specific testing based on each patient's posture and scapular position, rather than testing based on the pure frontal plane position of abduction).

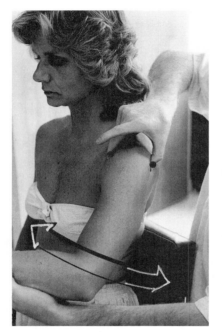

Patient Position: Patient sits.

Therapist Position: Therapist stands behind and to the side of the patient and cradles the patient's forearm with the elbow flexed with one hand. Therapist's other hand palpates the glenohumeral joint line. Therapist passively moves the patient's humerus aligning the extremity with the plane of the scapular spine. This position may involve a combined pattern of abduction with horizontal flexion or extension, depending on the specific posture of the patient's scapula.

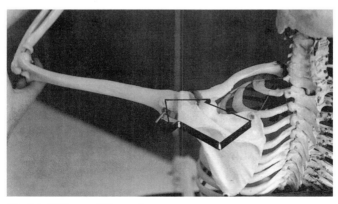

Skeletal Plane of Scapula

Glenohumeral

Abduction Overpressure

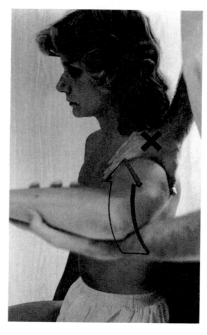

Patient Position: Patient sits or stands in neutral posture.

Therapist Position: Therapist stands behind the patient.

Stabilization: Therapist's medial hand stabilizes the scapula in an inferior direction (palm over the acromion).

Mobilization: Therapist's lateral hand cradles the patient's upper extremity (patient's elbow relaxed in flexion).

Direction of Force: Therapist's mobilizing hand abducts the shoulder to the end of range.

Glenohumeral

External Rotation Overpressure

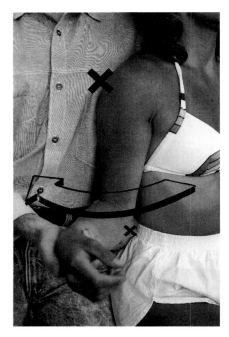

Patient Position: Patient sits or stands in neutral posture.

Therapist Position: Therapist stands behind the patient.

Stabilization: Therapist's medial hand stabilizes the elbow while the therapist's body provides stabilization of the patient's scapula.

Mobilization: Therapist's lateral hand grasps the patient's forearm (patient's elbow in 90° flexion).

Direction of Force: Therapist's mobilizing hand externally rotates the shoulder to the end of range.

Glenohumeral

Internal Rotation Overpressure

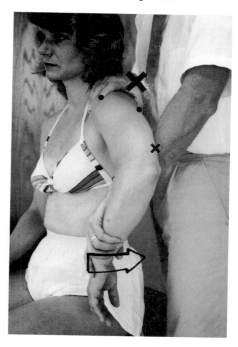

Patient Position: Patient sits or stands in neutral posture.

Therapist Position: Therapist stands behind the patient.

Stabilization: Therapist's medial hand stabilizes the scapula in an inferior direction (fingers over the coracoid process area and palm/forearm over the scapula).

Mobilization: Therapist's lateral hand grasps the patient's lower forearm (police-type hold) with the elbow in slight flexion.

Direction of Force: Therapist's mobilizing hand internally rotates the shoulder to the end of range.

Glenohumeral

"Functional" Position (Extension, Horizontal Adduction, and Internal Rotation) Overpressure

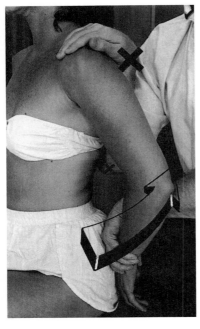

Patient Position: Patient sits or stands in neutral posture.

Therapist Position: Therapist stands behind the patient.

Stabilization: Therapist's medial hand stabilizes the scapula in an inferior direction (fingers over the coracoid process area and palm/forearm over the scapula).

Mobilization: Therapist's lateral hand grasps the patient's lower forearm (police-type hold) with the elbow in slight flexion.

Direction of Force: Therapist's mobilizing hand extends, adducts and internally rotates the shoulder (behind the back) to the end of range.

Glenohumeral

Horizontal Abduction Overpressure

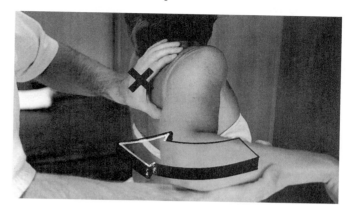

Patient Position: Patient sits or stands in neutral posture.

Therapist Position: Therapist stands behind the patient.

Stabilization: Therapist's medial hand stabilizes the scapula in an anterior and lateral direction.

Mobilization: Therapist's lateral hand grasps the patient's forearm with the elbow in flexion.

Direction of Force: Therapist's mobilizing hand horizontally abducts the shoulder to the end of range.

Glenohumeral

Horizontal Adduction Overpressure

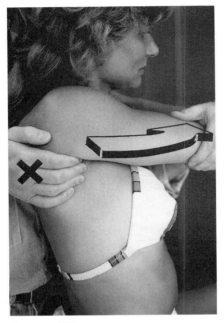

Patient Position: Patient sits or stands in neutral posture.

Therapist Position: Therapist stands behind the patient.

Stabilization: Therapist's lateral hand stabilizes the scapula in a posterior and medial direction (fingers grasp the lateral border of the scapula with the palm over the scapula).

Mobilization: Therapist's medial hand reaches in front of the patient and cradles the patient's upper extremity with the elbow in flexion.

Direction of Force: Therapist's mobilizing hand horizontally adducts the shoulder to the end of range.

Latereral View

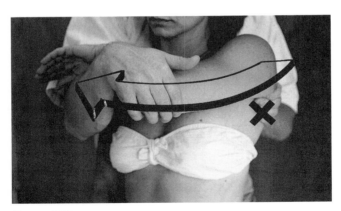

Frontal View

Elbow

Flexion Overpressure

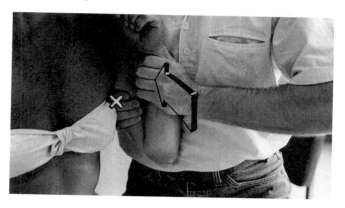

Patient Position: Patient sits or stands in neutral posture.

Therapist Position: Therapist stands alongside the patient's upper extremity.

Stabilization: Therapist's posterior hand stabilizes the humerus.

Mobilization: Therapist's anterior hand grasps the distal forearm.

Direction of Force: Therapist's mobilizing hand flexes the elbow to the end of range.

Elbow

Extension Overpressure

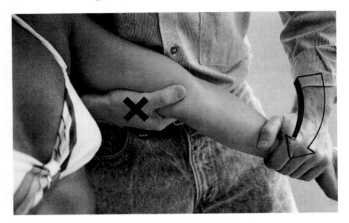

Patient Position: Patient sits or stands in neutral posture.

Therapist Position: Therapist stands alongside the patient's upper extremity.

Stabilization: Therapist's posterior hand stabilizes the humerus.

Mobilization: Therapist's anterior hand grasps the distal forearm.

Direction of Force: Therapist's mobilizing hand extends the elbow to the end of range.

Elbow/Forearm

Supination Overpressure

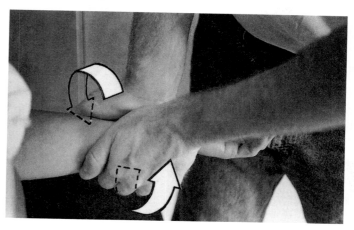

Patient Position: Patient sits or stands in neutral posture with the elbow flexed to 90°.

Therapist Position: Therapist faces the patient's upper extremity.

Stabilization: Therapist maintains the neutral position of the upper extremity.

Mobilization: Therapist's thenar eminence of the lateral hand grasps the patient's ventral radius and the therapist's fingers of the medial hand grasps the dorsal surface of the ulna.

Direction of Force: Therapist's hands simultaneously apply the mobilizing force in the direction of supination.

Elbow/Forearm

Pronation Overpressure

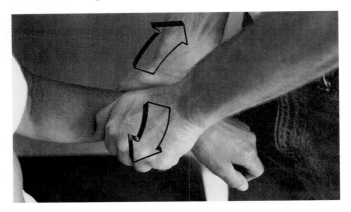

Patient Position: Patient sits or stands in neutral posture with the elbow flexed to 90°.

Therapist Position: Therapist faces the patient's upper extremity.

Stabilization: Therapist maintains the neutral position of the upper extremity.

Mobilization: Therapist's thenar eminence of the medial hand grasps the patient's dorsal radius and the therapist's fingers of the lateral hand grasp the ventral surface of the ulna.

Direction of Force: Therapist's hands simultaneously apply the mobilizing force in the direction of pronation.

Wrist

Flexion Overpressure

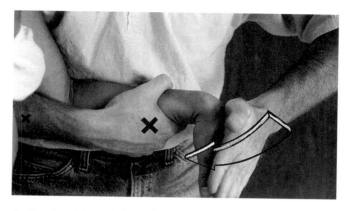

Patient Position: Patient sits or stands in neutral posture with the elbow in 90° flexion and/or full extension.

Therapist Position: Therapist stands alongside the patient's upper extremity.

Stabilization: Therapist's posterior hand stabilizes the patient's forearm.

Mobilization: Therapist's mobilization hand grasps the patient's hand dorsally.

Direction of Force: Therapist's mobilizing hand flexes the wrist to the end of range.

Wrist

Extension Overpressure

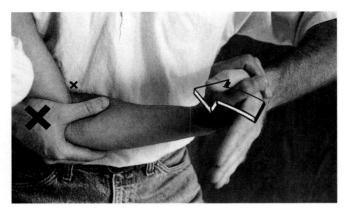

Patient Position: Patient sits or stands in neutral posture with the elbow in 90° flexion and/or full extension.

Therapist Position: Therapist stands alongside the patient's upper extremity.

Stabilization: Therapist's posterior hand stabilizes the patient's forearm.

Mobilization: Therapist's mobilization hand grasps the patient's hand on the palmar surface.

Direction of Force: Therapist's mobilizing hand extends the wrist to the end of range.

Wrist

Ulnar Deviation Overpressure

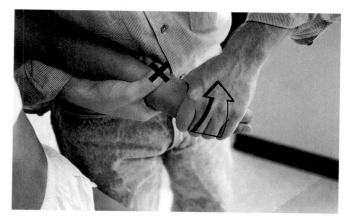

Patient Position: Patient sits or stands in neutral posture with the elbow in 90° flexion and/or full extension.

Therapist Position: Therapist stands alongside the patient's upper extremity.

Stabilization: Therapist's posterior hand stabilizes the patient's distal forearm. Therapist's body also provides stabilization.

Mobilization: Therapist's anterior hand grasps the radial side of the patient's hand.

Direction of Force: Therapist's mobilizing hand ulnarly deviates the wrist to the end of range.

Wrist

Radial Deviation Overpressure

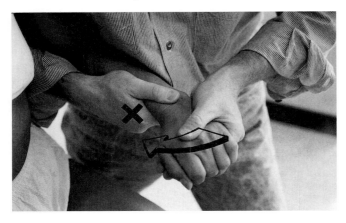

Patient Position: Patient sits or stands in neutral posture with the elbow in 90° flexion and/or full extension.

Therapist Position: Therapist stands alongside the patient's upper extremity.

Stabilization: Therapist's posterior hand stabilizes the patient's forearm. Therapist's body also provides stabilization.

Mobilization: Therapist's anterior hand grasps the ulnar side of the patient's hand.

Direction of Force: Therapist's mobilizing hand radially deviates the wrist to the end of range.

Finger

Flexion Overpressure

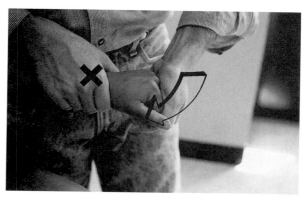

Group Finger Flexion Overpressure

Patient Position: Patient sits or stands in neutral posture with the elbow in 90° flexion and/or full extension and the wrist in neutral or in flexion.

Therapist Position: Therapist stands alongside the patient's upper extremity.

Stabilization: Therapist's posterior hand stabilizes the patient's wrist. Therapist's body also provides stabilization.

Mobilization: Therapist's anterior hand grasps the dorsal surface of the patient's fingers as a group or each finger individually.

Direction of Force: Therapist's mobilizing hand flexes the patient's fingers as a group or individually to the end of range.

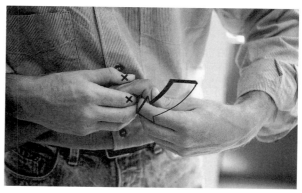

Individual Finger Flexion Overpressure

Finger

Extension Overpressure

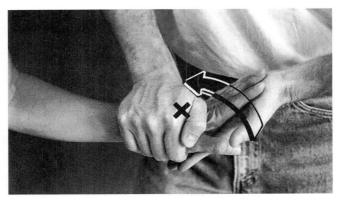

Group Finger Extension Overpressure

Patient Position: Patient sits or stands in neutral posture with the elbow in 90° flexion and/or full extension and the wrist in neutral or in extension.

Therapist Position: Therapist stands alongside the patient's upper extremity.

Stabilization: Therapist's posterior hand stabilizes the patient's wrist. Therapist's body also provides stabilization.

Mobilization: Therapist's anterior hand grasps the palmar surface of the patient's fingers as a group or each finger individually.

Direction of Force: Therapist's mobilizing hand extends the patient's fingers as a group or individually to the end of range.

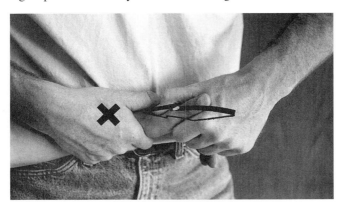

Thumb Extension Overpressure

Metacarpophalangeal I-V/Interphalangeal I-V

Distraction

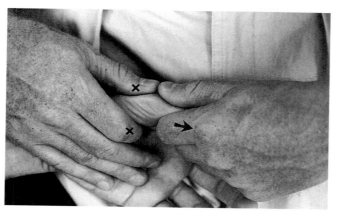

Thumb Metacarpophalangeal Distraction

Patient Position: Patient sits with the metacarpophalangeal (MCP) joint in slight flexion I-V and ulnar deviation II-V or the interphalangeal joint in slight flexion (LPP) with the forearm supported.

Therapist Position: Therapist stands alongside the patient's hand.

Stabilization: Therapist's proximal hand grasps the dorsal and volar surfaces of the distal end of the metacarpal.

Mobilization: Therapist's distal hand grasps the dorsal and volar surfaces of the proximal phalanx close to the MCP joint line.

Direction of Force: Therapist's mobilizing hand will distract the proximal phalanx on the metacarpal (figure above and bottom figure page 50).

Indication: Any capsular hypomobility.

The same technique is applied to all interphalangeal joints (top figure page 50).

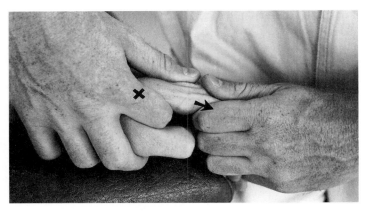

Interphalangeal Distraction

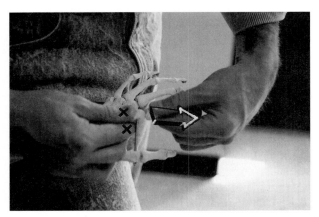

Skeletal Metacarpophalangeal Distraction

Metacarpophalangeal I-V/Interphalangeal I-V

Compression

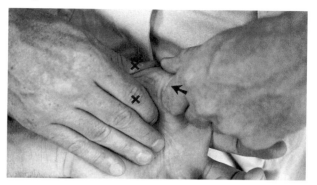

Thumb Metacarpophalangeal Compression

Patient Position: Patient sits with the metacarpophalangeal (MCP) joint in slight flexion I-V and ulnar deviation II-V or the interphalangeal joint in slight flexion (LPP) with the forearm supported.

Therapist Position: Therapist stands alongside the patient's hand.

Stabilization: Therapist's proximal hand grasps the dorsal and volar surfaces of the distal end of the metacarpal.

Mobilization: Therapist's distal hand grasps the dorsal and volar surfaces of the proximal phalanx at the MCP joint line.

Direction of Force: Therapist's mobilizing hand compresses the proximal phalanx into the metacarpal.

Indication: Provocation findings with arthritis.[1]

The same technique is applied to all interphalangeal joints.

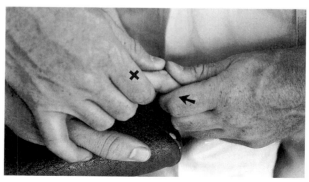

Interphalangeal Compression

Metacarpophalangeal I–V/Interphalangeal I–V

Dorsal Glide

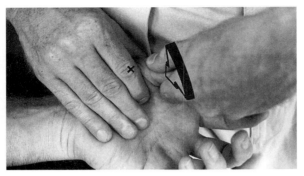

Thumb Metacarpophalangeal Dorsal Glide

Patient Position: Patient sits with the metacarpophalangeal (MCP) joint in slight flexion I–V and ulnar deviation II–V or the interphalangeal joint in slight flexion (LPP) with the forearm supported.

Therapist Position: Therapist stands alongside the patient's hand.

Stabilization: Therapist's proximal hand grasps the dorsal and volar surfaces of the distal end of the metacarpal.

Mobilization: Therapist's distal hand grasps the dorsal and volar surfaces of the proximal phalanx at the MCP joint line.

Direction of Force: Therapist's mobilizing hand glides the proximal phalanx dorsally on the metacarpal.

Indication: Extension hypomobility.

The same technique is applied to all interphalangeal joints.

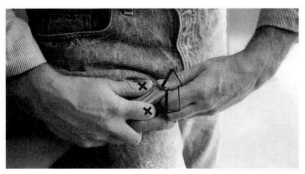

Interphalangeal Dorsal Glide

Metacarpophalangeal I–V/Interphalangeal I–V

Volar Glide

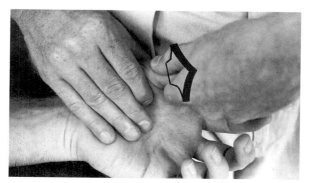

Thumb Metacarpophalangeal Volar Glide

Patient Position: Patient sits with the metacarpophalangeal (MCP) joint in slight flexion I–V and ulnar deviation II–V or the interphalangeal joint in slight flexion (LPP) with the forearm supported.

Therapist Position: Therapist stands alongside the patient's hand.

Stabilization: Therapist's proximal hand grasps the dorsal and volar surfaces of the distal end of the metacarpal.

Mobilization: Therapist's distal hand grasps the dorsal and volar surfaces of the proximal phalanx at the MCP joint line.

Direction of Force: Therapist's mobilizing hand glides the proximal phalanx volarly on the metacarpal.

Indication: Flexion hypomobility.

The same technique is applied to all interphalangeal joints.

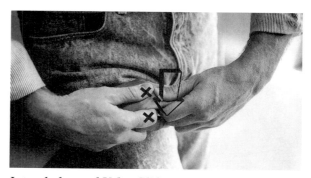

Interphalangeal Volar Glide

Metacarpophalangeal I–V/Interphalangeal I–V

Ulnar Glide

Patient Position: Patient sits with the metacarpophalangeal (MCP) joint in slight flexion I–V and ulnar deviation II–V or the interphalangeal joint in slight flexion (LPP) with the forearm supported. (See top figure, opposite page).

Therapist Position: Therapist stands alongside the patient's hand.

Stabilization: Therapist's proximal hand grasps the radial and ulnar surfaces of the distal end of the metacarpal.

Mobilization: Therapist's distal hand grasps the radial and ulnar surfaces of the proximal phalanx at the MCP joint line.

Direction of Force: Therapist's mobilizing hand glides the proximal phalanx ulnarly on the metacarpal.

Indications: Thumb flexion hypomobility, II & III ulnar deviation (adduction) hypomobility, and IV & V ulnar deviation (abduction) hypomobility.

The same technique is applied to all interphalangeal joints. (See bottom figure, opposite page).

Metacarpophalangeal I–V/Interphalangeal I–V

Ulnar Glide

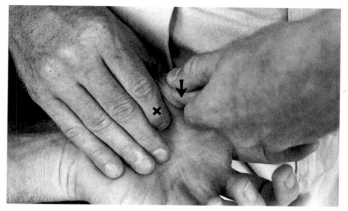

Thumb Metacarpophalangeal Ulnar Glide

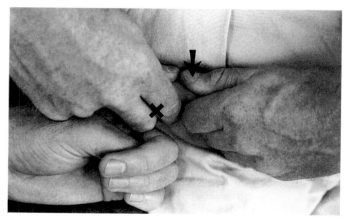

Interphalangeal Ulnar Glide

Metacarpophalangeal I–V/Interphalangeal I–V

Radial Glide

Patient Position: Patient sits with the metacarpophalangeal (MCP) joint in slight flexion I–V and ulnar deviation II–V or the interphalangeal joint in slight flexion (LPP) with the forearm supported (top figure, opposite page).

Therapist Position: Therapist stands alongside the patient's hand.

Stabilization: Therapist's proximal hand grasps the radial and ulnar surfaces of the distal end of the metacarpal.

Mobilization: Therapist's distal hand grasps the radial and ulnar surfaces of the proximal phalanx at the MCP joint line.

Direction of Force: Therapist's mobilizing hand glides the proximal phalanx radially on the metacarpal (top figure, opposite page).

Indications: Thumb extension hypomobility, II & III radial deviation (abduction) hypomobility, and IV & V radial deviation (adduction) hypomobility.

The same technique is applied to all interphalangeal joints (bottom figure, opposite page).

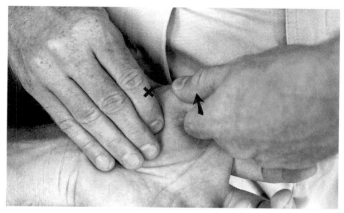

Thumb Metacarpophalangeal Radial Glide

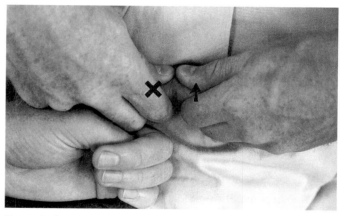

Interphalangeal Radial Glide

Metacarpophalangeal I–V/Interphalangeal I–V

Medial Rotation

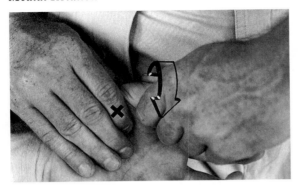

Thumb Metacarpophalangeal Medial Rotation

Patient Position: Patient sits with the metacarpophalangeal (MCP) joint in slight flexion I–V and ulnar deviation II–V or the interphalangeal joint in slight flexion (LPP) with the forearm supported.

Therapist Position: Therapist stands alongside the patient's hand.

Stabilization: Therapist's proximal hand grasps the radial and ulnar surfaces of the distal end of the metacarpal.

Mobilization: Therapist's distal hand grasps the radial and ulnar surfaces of the proximal phalanx at the MCP joint line.

Direction of Force: Therapist's mobilizing hand medially rotates the proximal phalanx on the metacarpal.

Indications: Thumb flexion hypomobility and II to V extension hypomobility.

The same technique is applied to all interphalangeal joints.

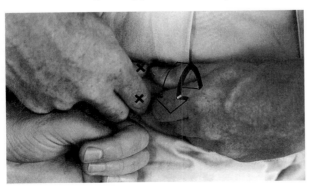

Interphalangeal Medial Rotation

Metacarpophalangeal I–V/Interphalangeal I–V

Lateral Rotation

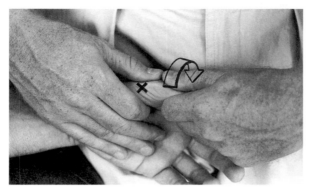

Thumb Metacarpophalangeal Lateral Rotation

Patient Position: Patient sits with the metacarpophalangeal (MCP) joint in slight flexion I–V and ulnar deviation II–V or the interphalangeal joint in slight flexion (LPP) with the forearm supported.

Therapist Position: Therapist stands alongside the patient's hand.

Stabilization: Therapist's proximal hand grasps the palmar and dorsal surfaces of the distal end of the metacarpal.

Mobilization: Therapist's distal hand grasps the palmar and dorsal surfaces of the proximal phalanx at the MCP joint line.

Direction of Force: Therapist's mobilizing hand laterally rotates the proximal phalanx on the metacarpal.

Indications: Thumb extension hypomobility and II to V flexion hypomobility.

The same technique is applied to all interphalangeal joints.

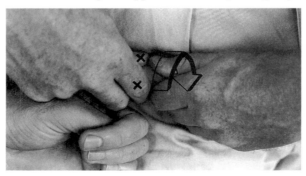

Interphalangeal Lateral Rotation

Carpometacarpal I

Distraction

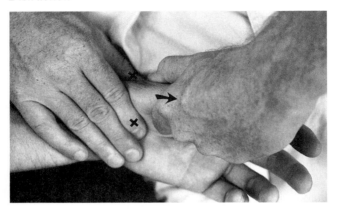

Patient Position: Patient sits with the thumb in neutral (LPP) and the forearm resting on the table.

Therapist Position: Therapist stands along the dorsal side of the patient's hand.

Stabilization: Therapist's proximal hand grasps the dorsal and volar surfaces of the trapezium.

Mobilization: Therapist's distal hand grasps the radial and ulnar surfaces of the first metacarpal.

Direction of Force: Therapist's mobilizing hand distracts the metacarpal from the trapezium in a distal direction.

Indication: Any capsular hypomobility.

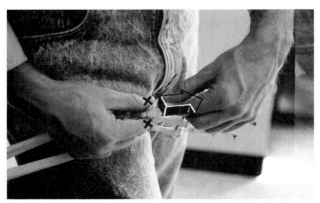

Skeletal Carpometacarpal I Distraction

Carpometacarpal I

Compression

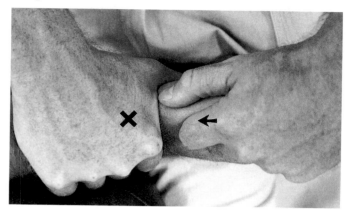

Patient Position: Patient sits with the thumb in neutral (LPP) and the forearm resting on the table.

Therapist Position: Therapist stands along the dorsal side of the patient's hand.

Stabilization: Therapist's proximal hand grasps the dorsal and volar surfaces of the trapezium.

Mobilization: Therapist's distal hand grasps the radial and ulnar surfaces of the first metacarpal.

Direction of Force: Therapist's mobilizing hand compresses the metacarpal into the trapezium in a proximal direction.

Indication: Provocation findings with arthritis.[1]

Carpometacarpal I

Dorsal Glide

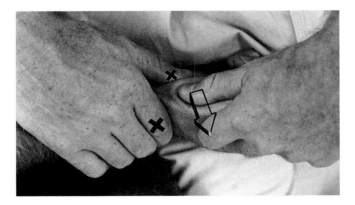

Patient Position: Patient sits with the thumb in neutral (LPP) and the forearm resting on the table.

Therapist Position: Therapist stands along the dorsal side of the patient's hand.

Stabilization: Therapist's proximal hand grasps the dorsal and volar surfaces of the trapezium.

Mobilization: Therapist's distal hand grasps the dorsal and volar surfaces of the first metacarpal at the joint line.

Direction of Force: Therapist's mobilizing hand glides the metacarpal in a dorsal direction on the trapezium.

Indication: Thumb abduction hypomobility.

Carpometacarpal I

Palmar/Volar Glide

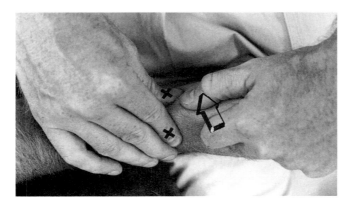

Patient Position: Patient sits with the thumb in neutral (LPP) and the forearm resting on the table.

Therapist Position: Therapist stands along the dorsal side of the patient's hand.

Stabilization: Therapist's proximal hand grasps around the dorsal and volar surfaces of the trapezium.

Mobilization: Therapist's distal hand grasps the dorsal and volar surfaces of the proximal portion of the first metacarpal at the joint line.

Direction of Force: Therapist's mobilizing hand glides the metacarpal in a palmar direction on the trapezium.

Indication: Thumb adduction hypomobility.

Carpometacarpal I

Ulnar Glide

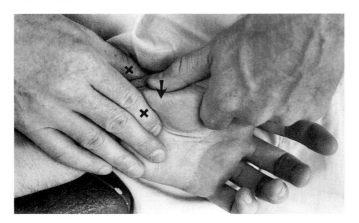

Patient Position: Patient sits with the thumb in neutral (LPP) and the forearm resting on the table.

Therapist Position: Therapist stands along the dorsal side of the patient's hand.

Stabilization: Therapist's proximal hand grasps the radial and ulnar surfaces of the trapezium.

Mobilization: Therapist's distal hand grasps the radial and ulnar surfaces of the first metacarpal at the joint line.

Direction of Force: Therapist's mobilizing hand glides the metacarpal in an ulnar direction on the trapezium.

Indication: Thumb flexion hypomobility.

Carpometacarpal I

Radial Glide

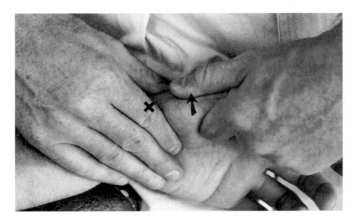

Patient Position: Patient sits with the thumb in neutral (LPP) and the forearm resting on the table.

Therapist Position: Therapist stands along the dorsal side of the patient's hand.

Stabilization: Therapist's proximal hand grasps the radial and ulnar surfaces of the trapezium.

Mobilization: Therapist's distal hand grasps the radial and ulnar surfaces of the proximal end of the first metacarpal at the joint line.

Direction of Force: Therapist's mobilizing hand glides the metacarpal in a radial direction on the trapezium.

Indication: Thumb extension hypomobility.

Carpometacarpal I

Medial Rotation

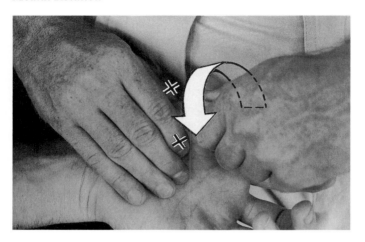

Patient Position: Patient sits with the thumb in neutral (LPP) and the forearm resting on the table.

Therapist Position: Therapist stands along the dorsal side of the patient's hand.

Stabilization: Therapist's proximal hand grasps the dorsal and volar surfaces of the trapezium.

Mobilization: Therapist's distal hand grasps the dorsal and volar surfaces of the first metacarpal at the joint line.

Direction of Force: Therapist's mobilizing hand rotates the metacarpal in a medial direction on the trapezium.

Indication: Thumb flexion hypomobility.

Carpometacarpal I

Lateral Rotation

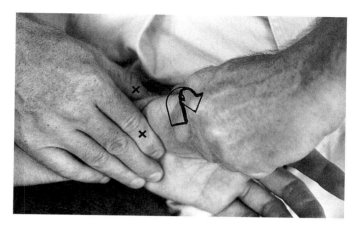

Patient Position: Patient sits with the thumb in neutral (LPP) and the forearm resting on the table.

Therapist Position: Therapist stands along the dorsal side of the patient's hand.

Stabilization: Therapist's proximal hand grasps the dorsal and volar surfaces of the trapezium.

Mobilization: Therapist's distal hand grasps the dorsal and volar surfaces of the first metacarpal at the joint line.

Direction of Force: Therapist's mobilizing hand rotates the metacarpal in a lateral direction on the trapezium.

Indication: Thumb extension hypomobility.

Intermetacarpal I–V

Dorsal Glide

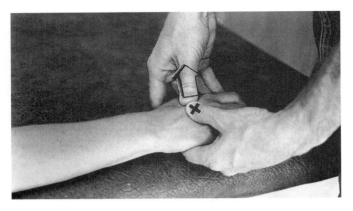

Patient Position: Patient sits with the wrist in neutral and the forearm resting on the table.

Therapist Position: Therapist stands facing the dorsal side of the patient's hand.

Stabilization: Therapist's hand grasps the dorsal surface of the metacarpals on the radial or ulnar side of the hand.

Mobilization: Therapist's other hand grasps the volar surface of the metacarpals on the opposing ulnar or radial side of the hand.

Direction of Force: Therapist's mobilizing hand glides the radial or ulnar metacarpals dorsally on the opposing ulnar or radial metacarpals.

Indications: I to V extension hypomobility.

Intermetacarpal I–V

Volar Glide

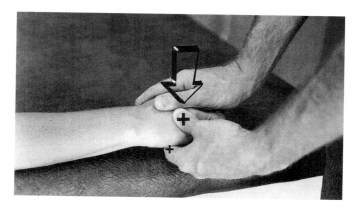

Patient Position: Patient sits with the wrist in neutral and the forearm resting on the table.

Therapist Position: Therapist stands facing the dorsal side of the patient's hand.

Stabilization: Therapist's hand grasps the volar surface of the metacarpals on the radial or ulnar side of the hand.

Mobilization: Therapist's other hand grasps the dorsal surface of the metacarpals on the opposing ulnar or radial side of the hand.

Direction of Force: Therapist's mobilizing hand glides the radial or ulnar metacarpals volarly on the opposing ulnar or radial metacarpals.

Indications: I to V flexion hypomobility.

Radiocarpal/Midcarpal

Distraction

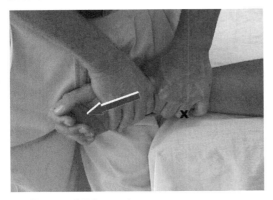

Radiocarpal Distraction

Patient Position: Patient sits with the wrist in slight flexion and ulnar deviation (LPP) with the forearm supported.

Therapist Position: Therapist stands alongside the patient's hand.

Stabilization: Therapist's proximal hand grasps the distal radius and ulna.

Mobilization: Therapist's distal hand grasps the proximal row of carpals (scaphoid, lunate, and triquetrum).

Direction of Force: Therapist's mobilizing hand distracts the proximal row of carpals in a volar/caudal/ulnar direction (both figures).

Indication: Any capsular hypomobility.

For the midcarpal joint, stabilize the proximal row of carpals and mobilize the distal row of carpals.

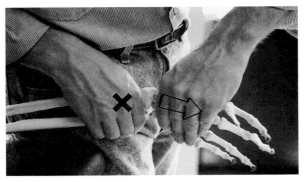

Skeletal Radiocarpal Distraction

Radiocarpal/Midcarpal

Compression

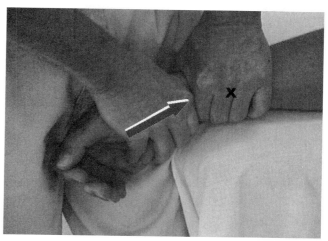

Radiocarpal Compression

Patient Position: Patient sits with the wrist in slight flexion and ulnar deviation (LPP) with the forearm supported.

Therapist Position: Therapist stands alongside the patient's hand.

Stabilization: Therapist's proximal hand grasps the distal radius and ulna.

Mobilization: Therapist's distal hand grasps the proximal row of carpals (scaphoid, lunate, and triquetrum) at the joint line.

Direction of Force: Therapist's mobilizing hand compresses the proximal row of carpals in a dorsal/cephalic/radial direction.

Indication: Provocation findings with arthritis.[1]

For the midcarpal joint, stabilize the proximal row of carpals and mobilize the distal row of carpals.

Radiocarpal/Midcarpal

Dorsal Glide

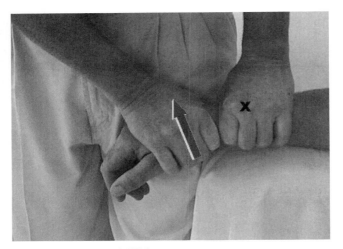

Radiocarpal Dorsal Glide

Patient Position: Patient sits with the wrist in slight flexion and ulnar deviation (LPP) with the forearm supported.

Therapist Position: Therapist stands alongside the patient's hand.

Stabilization: Therapist's proximal hand grasps the distal radius and ulna on the dorsal surface.

Mobilization: Therapist's distal hand grasps the palmar surface of the proximal row of carpals (scaphoid, lunate, and triquetrum) at the joint line.

Direction of Force: Therapist's mobilizing hand glides the proximal row of carpals in a dorsal caudal direction.

Indications: Wrist (especially the radiocarpal joint and the medial portion of the midcarpal joint) flexion hypomobility.

For the midcarpal joint, stabilize the proximal row of carpals and mobilize the distal row of carpals.

Radiocarpal/Midcarpal

Palmar/Volar Glide

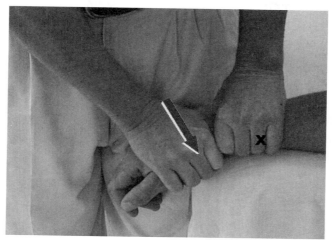

Radiocarpal Palmar/Volar Glide

Patient Position: Patient sits with the wrist in slight flexion and ulnar deviation (LPP) with the forearm supported.

Therapist Position: Therapist stands alongside the patient's hand.

Stabilization: Therapist's proximal hand grasps the volar surface of the distal radius and ulna.

Mobilization: Therapist's distal hand grasps the dorsal surface of the proximal row of carpals (scaphoid, lunate, and triquetrum) at the joint line.

Direction of Force: Therapist's mobilizing hand glides the proximal row of carpals in a palmar cephalic direction.

Indications: Wrist (especially the radiocarpal joint and the medial portion of the midcarpal joint) extension hypomobility.

For the midcarpal joint, stabilize the proximal row of carpals and mobilize the distal row of carpals.

Radiocarpal/Midcarpal

Ulnar Glide

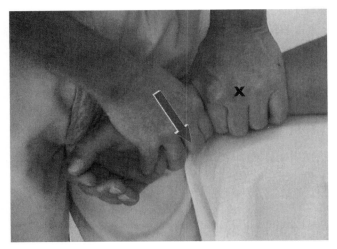

Radiocarpal Ulnar Glide

Patient Position: Patient sits with the wrist in slight flexion and ulnar deviation (LPP) with the forearm supported.

Therapist Position: Therapist stands alongside the patient's hand.

Stabilization: Therapist's proximal hand grasps the medial surface of the distal ulna.

Mobilization: Therapist's distal hand grasps the proximal row of carpals (scaphoid, lunate, and triquetrum).

Direction of Force: Therapist's mobilizing hand glides the proximal row of carpals in an ulnar cephalic direction.

Indications: Radiocarpal radial deviation hypomobility and midcarpal ulnar deviation hypomobility.

For the midcarpal joint, stabilize the proximal row of carpals and mobilize the distal row of carpals.

Radiocarpal/Midcarpal

Radial Glide

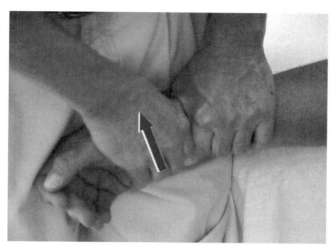

Radiocarpal Radial Glide

Patient Position: Patient sits with the wrist in slight flexion and ulnar deviation (LPP) with the forearm supported.

Therapist Position: Therapist stands alongside the patient's hand.

Stabilization: Therapist's proximal hand grasps the lateral surface of the distal radius.

Mobilization: Therapist's distal hand grasps the palmar surface of the proximal row of carpals (scaphoid, lunate, and triquetrum).

Direction of Force: Therapist's mobilizing hand glides the proximal row of carpals in a radial caudal direction.

Indications: Radiocarpal ulnar deviation hypomobility and midcarpal radial deviation hypomobility.

For the midcarpal joint, stabilize the proximal row of carpals and mobilize the distal row of carpals.

Radiocarpal/Midcarpal

Supination

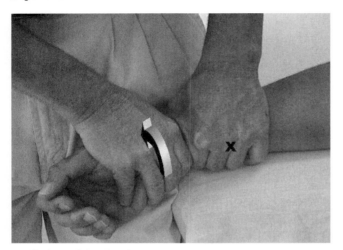

Radiocarpal Supination

Patient Position: Patient sits with the wrist in slight flexion and ulnar deviation (LPP) with the forearm supported.

Therapist Position: Therapist stands alongside the patient's hand.

Stabilization: Therapist's proximal hand grasps the distal radius and ulna.

Mobilization: Therapist's distal hand grasps the proximal row of carpals (scaphoid, lunate, and triquetrum).

Direction of Force: Therapist's mobilizing hand supinates the proximal row of carpals.

Indication: Supination hypomobility.

For the midcarpal joint, stabilize the proximal row of carpals and mobilize the distal row of carpals.

Radiocarpal/Midcarpal

Pronation

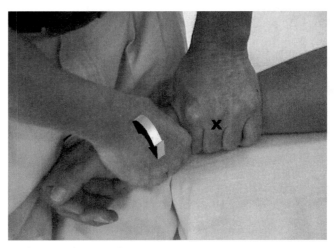

Radiocarpal Pronation

Patient Position: Patient sits with the wrist in slight flexion and ulnar deviation (LPP) with the forearm supported.

Therapist Position: Therapist stands alongside the patient's hand.

Stabilization: Therapist's proximal hand grasps the distal radius and ulna.

Mobilization: Therapist's distal hand grasps the proximal row of carpals (scaphoid, lunate, and triquetrum).

Direction of Force: Therapist's mobilizing hand pronates the proximal row of carpals.

Indication: Pronation hypomobility.

For the midcarpal joint, stabilize the proximal row of carpals and mobilize the distal row of carpals.

Distal Radioulnar

Compression

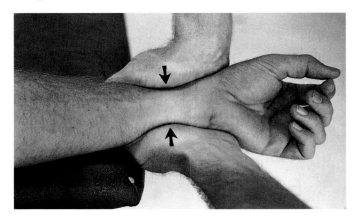

Patient Position: Patient sits with the forearm in 10° to 35° of supination.

Therapist Position: Therapist faces the patient.

Stabilization: The heel of one hand is placed over the distal ulna.

Mobilization: The heel of the other hand is placed over the distal radius.

Direction of Force: Therapist compresses the distal radius into the ulna.

Indication: Provocation finding with arthritis.[1]

Distal Radioulnar

Dorsal Glide

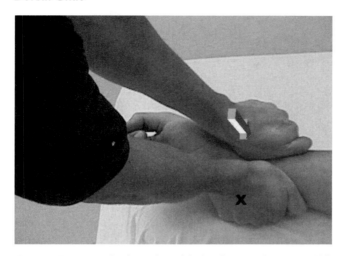

Patient Position: Patient sits with the forearm between 10° to 35° of supination (LPP).

Therapist Position: Therapist stands along the side to be mobilized.

Stabilization: Therapist's stabilization hand grasps the distal ulna using a lumbrical grip.

Mobilization: Therapist's mobilization hand grasps the distal radius using a lumbrical grip.

Direction of Force: Therapist's mobilizing hand glides the radius in a dorsal direction on the ulna.

Indication: Supination hypomobility.

Distal Radioulnar

Palmar/Volar Glide

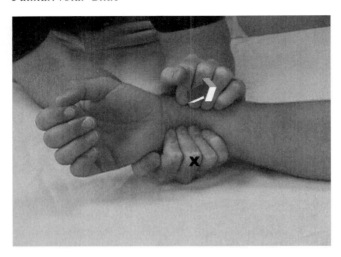

Patient Position: Patient sits with the forearm between 10° to 35° of supination (LPP).

Therapist Position: Therapist stands along the side to be mobilized.

Stabilization: Therapist's stabilization hand grasps the distal ulna using a lumbrical grip.

Mobilization: Therapist's mobilization hand grasps the distal radius using a lumbrical grip.

Direction of Force: Therapist's mobilizing hand glides the radius in a palmar/volar direction on the ulna.

Indication: Pronation hypomobility.

Humeroulnar

Distraction

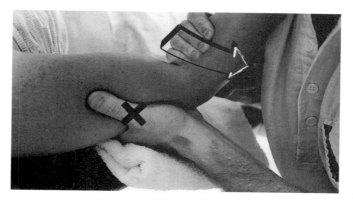

Patient Position: Patient lies supine with the elbow in 70° of flexion and between 10° to 35° of supination (LPP) with the upper arm resting on the table.

Therapist Position: Therapist faces the patient lateral to the forearm.

Stabilization: Therapist's lateral hand grasps the dorsal surface of the distal humerus.

Mobilization: Therapist's medial hand grasps the volar surface of the proximal ulna using a lumbrical grip.

Direction of Force: Therapist's mobilizing hand distracts the ulna in a caudal direction (direction of force is perpendicular to the plane of the ulna).

Indication: Any capsular hypomobility.

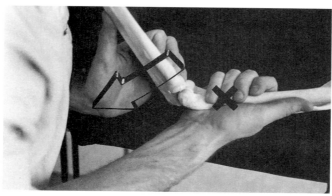

Skeletal Humeroulnar Distraction

Humeroulnar

Compression

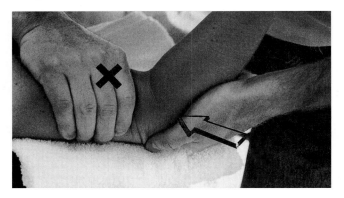

Patient Position: Patient lies supine with the elbow in 70° of flexion and be-tween 10° to 35° of supination (LPP) with the upper arm resting on the table.

Therapist Position: Therapist faces the patient lateral to the forearm.

Stabilization: Therapist's proximal hand grasps the volar surface of the distal humerus.

Mobilization: Therapist's distal hand grasps the dorsal surface of the proximal ulna.

Direction of Force: Therapist's mobilizing hand compresses in a cephalic direc-tion (direction of force is perpendicular to the plane of the ulna).

Indication: Provocation findings with arthritis.[1]

Humeroulnar

Cephalic Glide

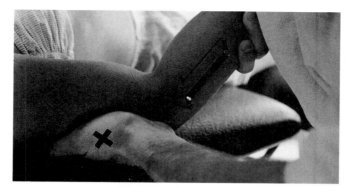

Patient Position: Patient lies supine with the elbow in 70° of flexion and 10° to 35° of supination (LPP) with the upper arm resting on the table.

Therapist Position: Therapist stands facing the patient's forearm.

Stabilization: Therapist's proximal hand supports the dorsal surface of the distal humerus.

Mobilization: Therapist's distal hand grasps the ulna using a lumbrical grip.

Direction of Force: Therapist's mobilizing hand glides the ulna cephalically through the long axis of the ulna.

Indications: Extension end range hypomobility, flexion end range hypomobility, and supination hypomobility.

Humeroulnar

Caudal Glide

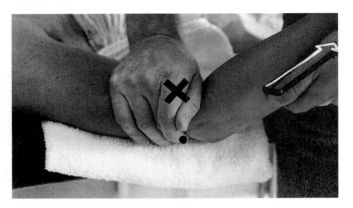

Patient Position: Patient lies supine with the elbow in 70° of flexion and 10° to 35° of supination (LPP) with the upper arm resting on the table.

Therapist Position: Therapist stands facing the patient's forearm.

Stabilization: Therapist's proximal hand grasps the anterior distal humerus.

Mobilization: Therapist's distal hand grasps the proximal ulna using a lumbrical grip.

Direction of Force: Therapist's mobilizing hand glides the ulna caudally through the long axis of the ulna.

Indications: Extension beginning range hypomobility, flexion beginning range hypomobility, and pronation hypomobility.

Humeroulnar/Humeroradial

Medial Tilt/Valgus Stress Test

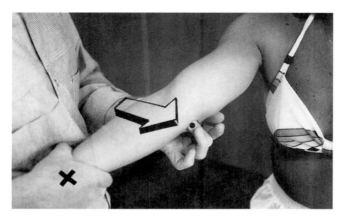

Patient Position: Patient sits with the elbow in full supination and just short of full extension.

Therapist Position: Therapist faces the patient along the side to be mobilized maintaining the patient's distal forearm against the therapist's body.

Stabilization: Therapist's distal hand grasps the distal radius and ulna maintaining the forearm in supination.

Mobilization: Therapist's proximal hand is placed over the lateral surface at the humeroradial joint line.

Direction of Force: Therapist's mobilizing hand pushes from a lateral to medial direction. One finger of the mobilization hand palpates the medial movement of the olecranon.

Indications: Humeroulnar extension hypomobility and supination hypomobility; and medial collateral ligament involvement with stress testing.

Humeroulnar/Humeroradial

Lateral Tilt/Varus Stress Test

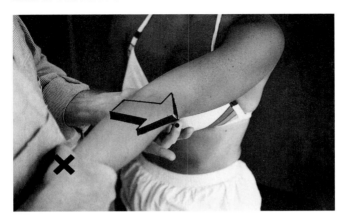

Patient Position: Patient sits with the elbow in full supination and just short of full extension.

Therapist Position: Therapist stands between the patient and the arm facing laterally, maintaining the patient's distal forearm against the therapist's body.

Stabilization: Therapist's distal hand grasps the distal radius and ulna maintaining the forearm in supination.

Mobilization: Therapist's proximal hand is placed over the medial surface at the humeroulnar joint line.

Direction of Force: Therapist's mobilizing hand pushes from a medial to lateral direction. One finger of the mobilization hand palpates the lateral movement of the olecranon and/or gapping of the humeroradial joint.

Indications: Humeroulnar flexion hypomobility and pronation hypomobility; lateral collateral ligament involvement with stress testing.

Humeroradial

Distraction

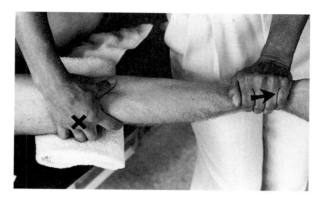

Patient Position: Patient lies supine with the shoulder in abduction and the elbow in full extension and supination (LPP).

Therapist Position: Therapist stands inside the arm and faces the patient's forearm.

Stabilization: Therapist's proximal hand grasps the anterolateral surface of the distal humerus and palpates the humeroradial joint line.

Mobilization: Therapist's distal hand grasps the distal radius using a lumbrical grip.

Direction of Force: Therapist's mobilizing hand distracts the radius through the long axis of the radius in a caudal direction.

Indication: Any capsular hypomobility.

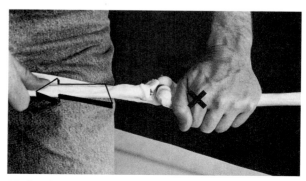

Skeletal Humeroradial Distraction

Humeroradial

Compression

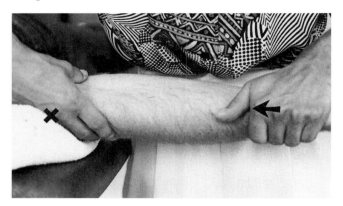

Patient Position: Patient lies supine with the shoulder in abduction and the elbow in full extension and supination (LPP).

Therapist Position: Therapist stands inside the arm and faces the patient's forearm.

Stabilization: Therapist's proximal hand grasps the anterolateral surface of the distal humerus and palpates the humeroradial joint line.

Mobilization: Therapist's distal hand grasps the distal radius using a lumbrical grip.

Direction of Force: Therapist's mobilizing hand compresses the radius through the long axis of the radius in a cephalic direction.

Indication: Provocation finding with arthritis.[1]

Humeroradial

Dorsal Glide

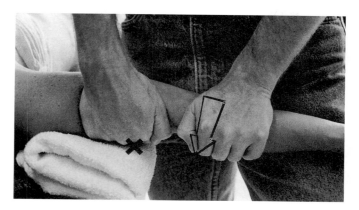

Patient Position: Patient lies supine with the shoulder in abduction and the elbow in full extension and supination (LPP).

Therapist Position: Therapist stands inside the arm and faces the patient's forearm.

Stabilization: The table, towel, and therapist's proximal hand provide stabilization of the humerus close to the joint line.

Mobilization: Therapist's distal hand is placed with the thenar eminence over the anterior radial head.

Direction of Force: Therapist's mobilizing hand glides the radius in a dorsal direction perpendicular to the humerus.

Indication: Extension hypomobility.

Humeroradial

Palmar/Volar Glide

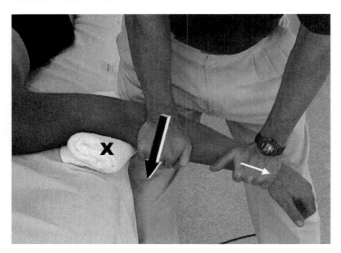

Patient Position: Patient lies prone with the shoulder in abduction, the humerus resting on the table, and the elbow in full extension and supination (LPP).

Therapist Position: Therapist stands inside the arm facing the patient's forearm.

Stabilization: The table, towel, and therapist's proximal hand provide stabilization of the humerus close to the joint line.

Mobilization: Therapist's distal hand using the thenar eminence is placed over the posterior radial head.

Direction of Force: Therapist's mobilizing hand glides the humerus in a palmar/volar direction perpendicular to the humerus.

Indication: Flexion hypomobility.

Humeroradial

Rotation

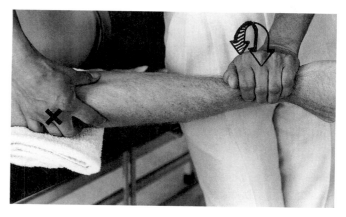

Patient Position: Patient lies supine with the elbow in full extension and the forearm in supination.

Therapist Position: Therapist stands inside the arm and faces the patient's forearm.

Stabilization: Therapist's proximal hand grasps the anterolateral surface of the distal humerus and palpates at the humeroradial joint line.

Mobilization: Therapist's distal hand grasps the distal radius proximal to the radiocarpal joint using a lumbrical grip.

Direction of Force: Therapist's mobilizing hand pronates and/or supinates the forearm.

Indications: Pronation hypomobility or supination hypomobility.

Proximal Radioulnar

Dorsal Glide

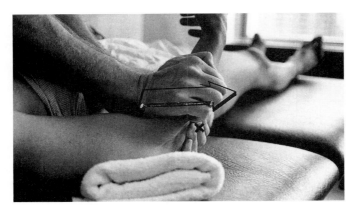

Patient Position: Patient sits or lies supine with the elbow in 70° of flexion and between 10° to 35° of supination (LPP).

Therapist Position: Therapist stands on the opposite side to be mobilized reaching across the patient.

Stabilization: Therapist's proximal hand grasps under the proximal ulna on the dorsal side.

Mobilization: Therapist's distal hand grasps the radial head with the heel of the hand on the volar side, forearm parallel to the direction of movement.

Direction of Force: Therapist's mobilizing hand glides the radius in a dorsal direction on the ulna.

Indication: Pronation hypomobility.

Proximal Radioulnar

Volar Glide

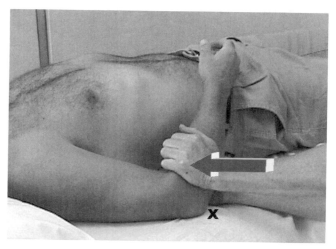

Patient Position: Patient sits or lies supine with the elbow in 70° of flexion and 10° to 35° of supination (LPP) with the forearm resting on the table or on the patient.

Therapist Position: Therapist stands on the side to be mobilized facing the patient.

Stabilization: Therapist's stabilization hand grasps the proximal ulna with a lumbrical grip.

Mobilization: Therapist's mobilization hand grasps the radial head with the heel of the hand on the dorsal surface, forearm parallel to the direction of movement.

Direction of Force: Therapist's mobilizing hand glides the radius in a volar direction on the ulna (figure above).

Indication: Supination hypomobility.

Proximal Radioulnar

Cephalic Glide

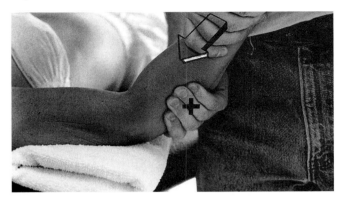

Patient Position: Patient lies supine with the elbow in 70° of flexion and between 10° to 35° of supination (LPP).

Therapist Position: Therapist stands inside the arm and faces the patient's forearm.

Stabilization: Therapist's stabilization hand grasps the proximal ulna with a lumbrical grip.

Mobilization: Therapist's mobilization hand grasps the distal radius with a lumbrical grip.

Direction of Force: Therapist's mobilizing hand glides the radius cephalically. The motion occurs simultaneously at both the proximal and distal radioulnar joints.

Indication: Pronation hypomobility.

Proximal Radioulnar

Caudal Glide

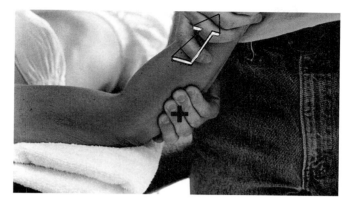

Patient Position: Patient lies supine with the elbow in 70° of flexion and between 10° to 35° of supination (LPP).

Therapist Position: Therapist stands inside the arm and faces the patient's forearm.

Stabilization: Therapist's proximal hand grasps the ulna with a lumbrical grip.

Mobilization: Therapist's distal hand grasps the distal radius with a lumbrical grip.

Direction of Force: Therapist's mobilizing hand glides the radius in a caudal direction. The motion occurs simultaneously at both the proximal and distal radioulnar joints.

Indication: Supination hypomobility.

Proximal Radioulnar

Rotation

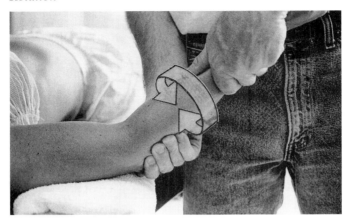

Patient Position: Patient lies supine with the elbow in 70° of flexion and between 10° to 35° of supination (LPP).

Therapist Position: Therapist stands inside the arm and faces the patient's forearm.

Stabilization: Therapist's proximal hand grasps the anterolateral surface of the proximal ulna and a finger palpates the radial head.

Mobilization: Therapist's distal hand grasps the distal radius using a lumbrical grip.

Direction of Force: Therapist's mobilizing hand rotates the radius into pronation and/or supination.

Indications: Pronation hypomobility or supination hypomobility.

Glenohumeral

Lateral Distraction

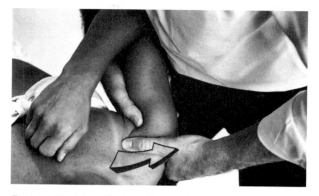

Patient Position: Patient lies supine with the glenohumeral joint line over the edge of the table. The humerus is in 55° of abduction and 30° of horizontal adduction (LPP) and the elbow flexed to a relaxed position.

Therapist Position: Therapist faces the patient's shoulder, cradling the extremity in the LPP between the distal arm and trunk.

Stabilization: Therapist's proximal hand is placed with the thumb over the coracoid process and the rest of the hand over the superior and posterior scapula.

Mobilization: Therapist's distal hand is placed in the axilla at the proximal medial portion of the humerus.

Direction of Force: Therapist's mobilizing hand distracts in a superior, lateral, and anterior direction (by the therapist leaning back).

Indication: Any capsular hypomobility.

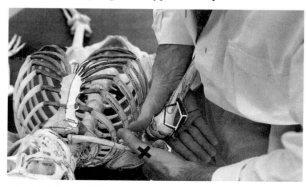

Skeletal Lateral Distraction

Glenohumeral

Compression

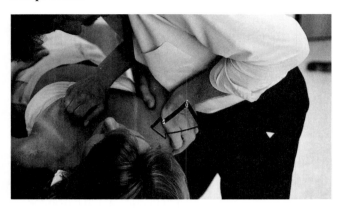

Patient Position: Patient lies supine with the glenohumeral joint line over the edge of the table. The humerus is in 55° of abduction and 30° of horizontal adduction (LPP) and the elbow flexed to a relaxed position.

Therapist Position: Therapist faces the patient's shoulder, cradling the extremity in the LPP between the caudal arm and trunk.

Stabilization: The scapula is stabilized by the table and the patient's thoracic wall.

Mobilization: Therapist's proximal hand is placed with the heel over the superior and lateral portion of the proximal humerus.

Direction of Force: Therapist's mobilizing hand compresses the humerus in an inferior, medial, and posterior direction into the scapula.

Indication: Provocation findings with arthritis.[1]

Glenohumeral

Anterior Glide

Patient Position: Patient lies prone with the glenohumeral joint line over the edge of the table. The humerus is in 55° of abduction and 30° of horizontal adduction (LPP) and the elbow flexed to a relaxed position.

Therapist Position: Therapist stands between the patient's trunk and extremity, placing the therapist's thigh close to the patient's axilla. Therapist supports the patient's arm in the LPP with the therapist's caudal arm.

Stabilization: The scapula is stabilized by the table and/or with a towel/wedge placed under the coracoid process anteriorly.

Mobilization: Therapist's proximal hand is placed with the heel over the proximal posterior area of the humeral head. The therapist's fingers extend around the anterior humeral head to palpate the movement (and to return the humerus to the neutral position if necessary). Piccolo distraction prior to mobilization is provided by the therapist's cephalic leg moving the humerus laterally.

Direction of Force: Therapist's mobilizing hand and body glide the humerus in an anterior, medial, and inferior direction.

Indications: Flexion end range hypomobility, extension hypomobility, external rotation hypomobility, and horizontal abduction hypomobility.

Glenohumeral

Anterior Glide

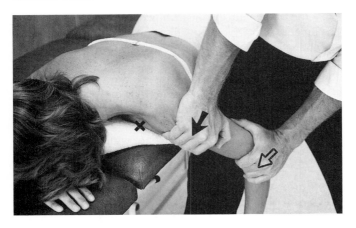

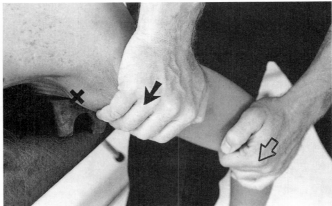

Anterior Glide with Wedge

Glenohumeral

Posterior Glide

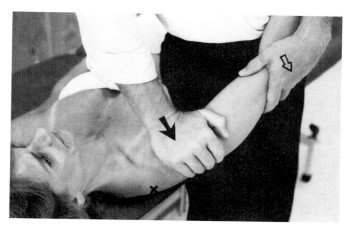

Patient Position: Patient lies supine with the glenohumeral joint line over the edge of the table. The humerus is in 55° of abduction and 30° of horizontal adduction (LPP) and the elbow flexed to a relaxed position.

Therapist Position: Therapist stands between the patient's trunk and extremity, placing the therapist's thigh close to the patient's axilla. Therapist supports the patient's arm in the LPP with the therapist's caudal arm.

Stabilization: The scapula is stabilized by the table and/or with a towel/wedge placed posteriorly.

Mobilization: Therapist's proximal hand is placed with the heel over the anterior and proximal area of the humeral head. The therapist's fingers extend around the posterior humeral head to palpate the movement (and to return the humerus to the neutral position if necessary). Piccolo distraction prior to mobilization is provided by the therapist's cephalic leg moving the humerus laterally.

Direction of Force: Therapist's mobilizing hand and body glide the humerus in a posterior, lateral, and superior direction.

Indications: Flexion hypomobility, internal rotation hypomobility, and horizontal adduction hypomobility.

Glenohumeral

Inferior Glide without Stabilization

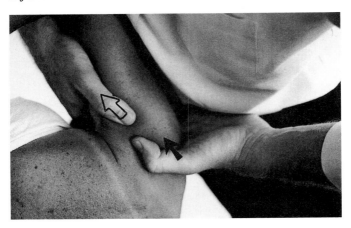

Patient Position: Patient lies supine with the shoulder in 55° of abduction and 30° of horizontal adduction (LPP) and the elbow flexed to a relaxed position.

Therapist Position: Therapist faces the patient's shoulder, cradling the extremity in the LPP between the caudal arm and trunk.

Stabilization: Provided by the patient's body weight.

Mobilization: Therapist's distal hand grasps the proximal medial humerus in the axilla providing piccolo distraction in a superior, lateral, and anterior direction relative to the scapula. Therapist's proximal hand is placed just lateral to the acromion with the web space over the superior humeral head.

Direction of Force: Therapist's mobilizing hand glides the humerus inferiorly by shifting the therapist's body in a caudal direction.

Indications: Abduction hypomobility, flexion hypomobility, and extension hypomobility.

Glenohumeral

Inferior Glide with Stabilization

Patient Position: Patient lies supine with the shoulder in 55° of abduction and 30° of horizontal adduction (LPP) and the elbow flexed to a relaxed position.

Therapist Position: Therapist faces the patient's shoulder, cradling the extremity in the LPP between the caudal arm and trunk.

Stabilization: Therapist's distal hand (dorsal surface) is placed into the patient's axilla. The neck of the scapula is grasped within the web space of the hand to stabilize the scapula (figure at bottom of page 104).

Mobilization: Therapist's proximal hand is placed just lateral to the tip of the acromion with the web space over the superior humeral head.

Direction of Force: Therapist's mobilizing hand glides the humerus inferiorly by shifting the therapist's body in a caudal direction (figure at top of page 104).

Indications: Abduction hypomobility, flexion hypomobility, and extension hypomobility.

Glenohumeral

Inferior Glide with Stabilization

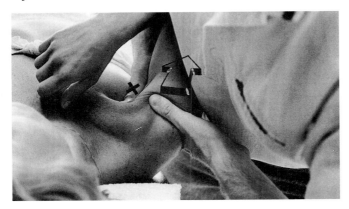

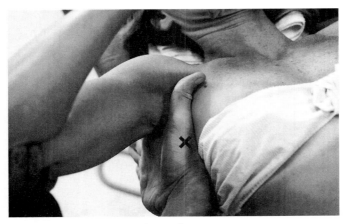

Stabilization with Web of Hand

Subacromial

Long Axis Distraction

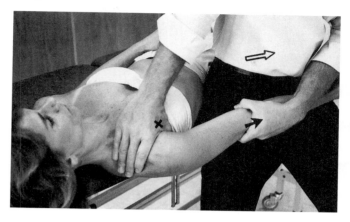

Patient Position: Patient lies supine with the humerus over the edge of the table in the anatomic position (LPP) with the elbow flexed to a relaxed position.

Therapist Position: Therapist stands between the patient's trunk and extremity, maintaining the extremity in the anatomic position (LPP).

Stabilization: Therapist's proximal hand is placed in the patient's axilla with the thumb under the neck of the scapula and the fingers over the coracoid process.

Mobilization: Therapist's distal hand grasps the distal humerus.

Direction of Force: Therapist shifts his/her body weight, distracting the sub-acromial joint in a caudal direction.

Indications: Subacromial impingement and inferior glenohumeral capsular hypomobility.

Subacromial

Long Axis Compression

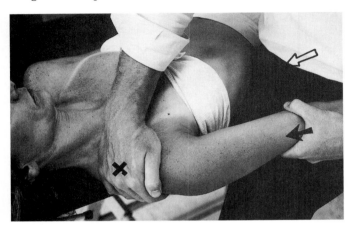

Patient Position: Patient lies supine with the humerus over the edge of the table in the anatomic position (LPP) with the elbow flexed to a relaxed position.

Therapist Position: Therapist stands between the patient's trunk and extremity, maintaining the extremity in the anatomic position (LPP).

Stabilization: Therapist's proximal hand is placed over the superior part of the acromion.

Mobilization: Therapist's distal hand grasps the distal humerus.

Direction of Force: Therapist shifts his/her body weight, compressing the sub-acromial joint in a cephalic direction.

Indication: Provocation findings with subacromial impingement.

Acromioclavicular (AC)

Active Movement Testing

Patient Position: Patient sits.

Therapist Position: Therapist stands behind the patient.

Stabilization: Provided by the patient's body weight.

Mobilization: Therapist palpates the AC joint lines bilaterally.

Direction of Force: Patient actively elevates (figure A below), depresses (figure B below), protracts (figure A page 108), and retracts (figure B page 108) the shoulder girdle slowly.

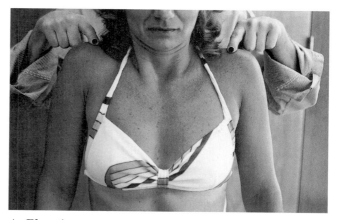

A: Elevation

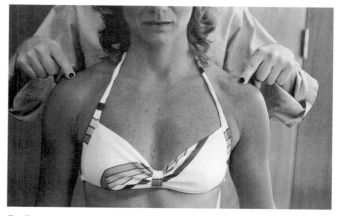

B: Depression

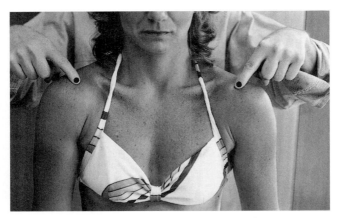

A: Protraction

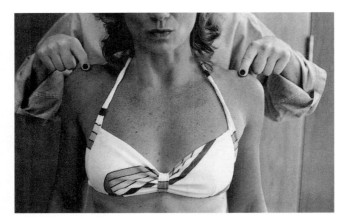

B: Retraction

Acromioclavicular

Distraction/Anterior Glide

Patient Position: Patient lies supine with the shoulder girdle in the anatomic position (LPP) near the edge of the table. (See figures on next page).

Therapist Position: Therapist stands on the side to be mobilized at the head of the patient.

Stabilization: Therapist's stabilization force is through the fingers of the laterally placed hand over the anterior acromion.

Mobilization: Therapist uses both thumbs placed alongside one another, or one over another, on the posterior lateral clavicle close to the joint line.

Direction of Force: For distraction, the therapist's mobilizing force is through the thumbs directed in an anterior medial direction (see figures on next page). For an anterior glide, the force is in an anterior lateral direction.

Indication: Distraction for any capsular hypomobility; anterior glide for protraction hypomobility.

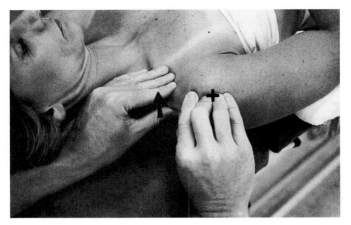

Acromioclavicular Distraction

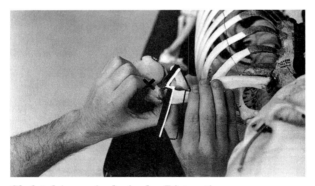

Skeletal Acromioclavicular Distraction

Acromioclavicular

Compression/Posterior Glide

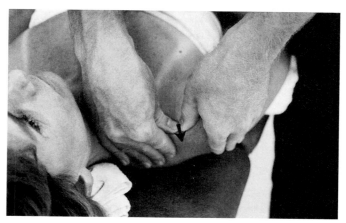

Acromioclavicular Compression

Patient Position: Patient lies supine with the shoulder girdle in the anatomic position (LPP) near the edge of the table.

Therapist Position: Therapist stands facing the patient's head.

Stabilization: Therapist's stabilization force is through the fingers of the laterally placed hand along the posterior acromion.

Mobilization: Therapist uses both thumbs placed alongside one another, or one over another, on the anterior lateral clavicle close to the joint line.

Direction of Force: For compression, the therapist's mobilizing force is through the thumbs directed in a posterior lateral direction. For a posterior glide, the force is in a posterior medial direction.

Indication: Compression for provocation findings with arthritis;[1] posterior glide for retraction hypomobility.

Acromioclavicular

Cephalic/Caudal Glide (Acromion on Clavicle)

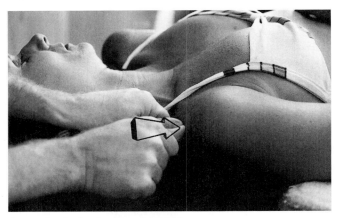

Acromioclavicular Caudal Glide

Patient Position: Patient lies supine with the upper extremity in the neutral position.

Therapist Position: Therapist stands at the patient's head on the side to be tested.

Stabilization: Provided by the patient's body weight.

Mobilization: Therapist places the pads (or tips) of both thumbs on the acromion (caudal glide) or clavicle (relative cephalic glide).

Direction of Force: Therapist glides the acromion or clavicle in a caudal direction that produces a caudal or relative cephalic motion (respectively) of the acromion on the clavicle.

Indication: Cephalic for elevation hypomobility; caudal for depression hypomobility.

Sternoclavicular (SC)

Active Movement Testing

Patient Position: Patient sits.

Therapist Position: Therapist stands behind the patient.

Stabilization: Provided by the patient's body weight.

Mobilization: Therapist palpates the SC joint lines bilaterally.

Direction of Force: Patient actively elevates (figure A below), depresses (figure B below), protracts (figure A page 114), and retracts (figure B page 114) the shoulder girdle slowly.

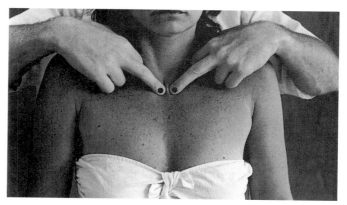

A: Elevation

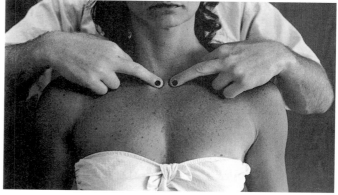

B: Depression

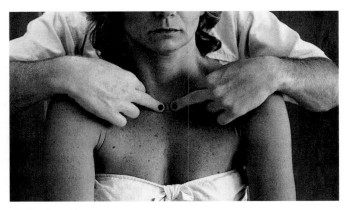

A: Protraction

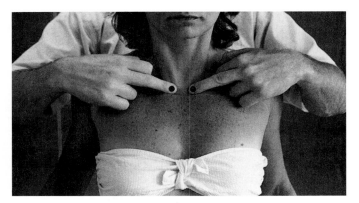

B: Retraction

Sternoclavicular

Distraction

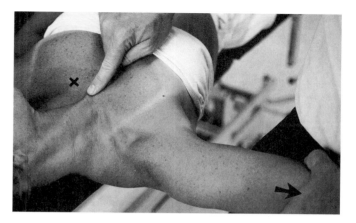

Patient Position: Patient lies supine with the humerus abducted to form a horizontal line with the clavicle. The patient's elbow is flexed.

Therapist Position: Therapist stands between the patient's extremity and trunk.

Stabilization: Provided by the patient's body weight.

Mobilization: Therapist grasps the patient's upper extremity at the distal humerus, while the other hand palpates the SC joint line.

Direction of Force: Therapist distracts the SC joint by leaning away from the patient in a lateral direction.

Indication: Any capsular hypomobility.

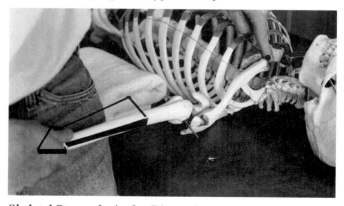

Skeletal Sternoclavicular Distraction

Sternoclavicular

Compression

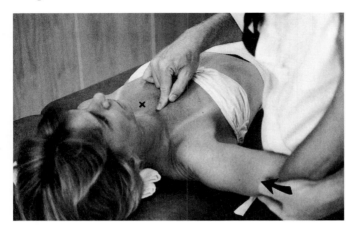

Patient Position: Patient lies supine with the humerus abducted to form a horizontal line with the clavicle. The patient's elbow is flexed.

Therapist Position: Therapist stands between the patient's extremity and trunk.

Stabilization: Provided by the patient's body weight.

Mobilization: Therapist grasps the patient's upper extremity at the distal humerus.

Direction of Force: Therapist compresses the SC joint by leaning toward the patient in a medial direction.

Indication: Provocation finding with arthritis.[1]

Sternoclavicular

Anterior Glide

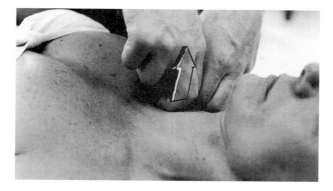

Patient Position: Patient lies supine with the shoulder girdle in the anatomic position (LPP).

Therapist Position: Therapist stands on either side of the patient.

Stabilization: Provided by the patient's body weight.

Mobilization: Therapist's index fingers pull the clavicle anteriorly from the medial end of the clavicle (figure above) or the anterior return movement of the clavicle following a posterior glide of the clavicle on the sternum (figure below) is used as an anterior glide. The therapist assesses both the quantity and quality of the return movement.

Direction of Force: The clavicle glides anteriorly and medially on the sternum.

Indication: Protraction hypomobility.

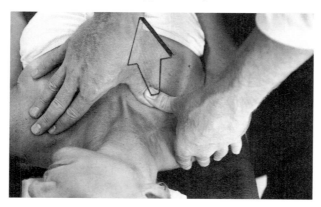

Sternoclavicular

Posterior Glide

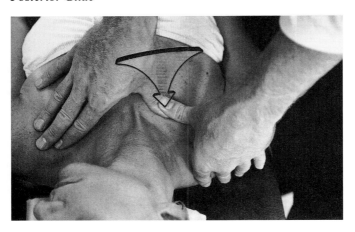

Patient Position: Patient lies supine with the shoulder girdle in the anatomic position (LPP).

Therapist Position: Therapist stands on either side of the patient.

Stabilization: Provided by the patient's body weight.

Mobilization: Therapist's two thumbs are placed over the anterior surface of the medial end of the clavicle.

Direction of Force: Therapist glides the clavicle on the sternum in a posterior and lateral direction.

Indication: Retraction hypomobility.

Sternoclavicular

Superior Glide

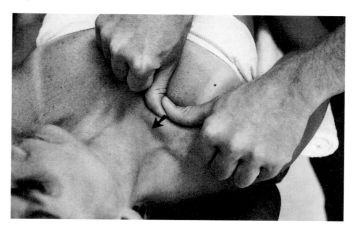

Patient Position: Patient lies supine with the shoulder girdle in the anatomic position (LPP) near the edge of the table.

Therapist Position: Therapist stands facing the head of the patient.

Stabilization: Provided by the patient's body weight.

Mobilization: Therapist's two thumbs are placed over the inferior surface of the medial end of the clavicle.

Direction of Force: Therapist glides the clavicle on the sternum in a superior and medial direction.

Indication: Depression hypomobility.

Sternoclavicular

Inferior Glide

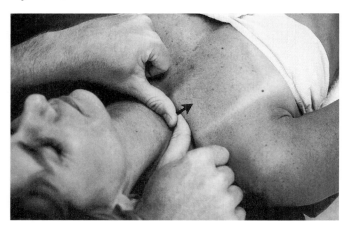

Patient Position: Patient lies supine with the shoulder girdle in the anatomic position (LPP) near the edge of the table.

Therapist Position: Therapist stands at the head of the patient.

Stabilization: Provided by the patient's body weight.

Mobilization: Therapist's two thumbs are placed over the superior surface of the medial end of the clavicle.

Direction of Force: Therapist glides the clavicle on the sternum in an inferior and lateral direction.

Indication: Elevation hypomobility.

Scapulothoracic

Distraction

Patient Position: Patient lies prone or is side-lying with the shoulder girdle in the anatomic position (LPP) (see figures on next page). In prone, the patient's hand is placed in the small of the back. In side-lying, the patient's upper arm rests on the lateral chest wall.

Therapist Position: With the patient prone, the therapist stands along the side to be mobilized facing the patient. The therapist's cephalic arm cradles the patient's upper extremity. With the patient side-lying, the therapist faces the patient with the therapist's caudal hand resting under the patient's arm.

Stabilization: Provided by the patient's body weight.

Mobilization: With the patient prone or side-lying, the therapist's cephalic hand supports the scapula anteriorly at the coracoid process; the caudal hand grasps under the medial border of the scapula.

Direction of Force: Therapist's hands distract the scapula in a perpendicular direction, away from the thoracic wall.

Indication: Any capsular hypomobility.

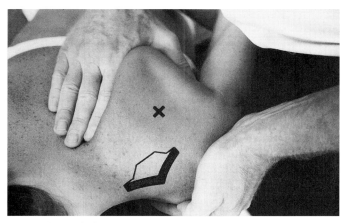

Prone Scapulothoracic Distraction

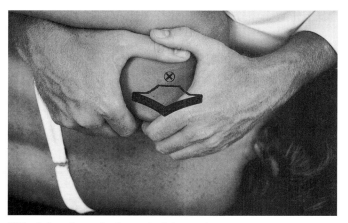

Side-lying Scapulothoracic Distraction

Scapulothoracic

Superior Glide

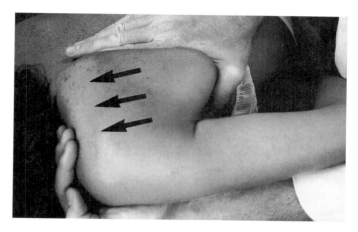

Patient Position: Patient lies prone or is side-lying, with the shoulder girdle in the anatomic position (LPP). (a) In prone, the patient's hand is placed in the small of the back. (b) In side-lying, the patient's upper arm rests on the lateral chest wall.

Therapist Position: (a) With the patient prone, the therapist stands along the side to be mobilized facing the patient. The therapist's cephalic arm cradles the patient's upper extremity. (b) With the patient side-lying, the therapist faces the patient with the therapist's caudal hand resting under the patient's arm.

Stabilization: Provided by the patient's body weight.

Mobilization: With the patient prone or side-lying, the therapist's cephalic hand supports the scapula anteriorly at the coracoid process; the caudal hand grasps under the medial border of the scapula.

Direction of Force: Therapist's hands glide the scapula superiorly along the thoracic wall.

Indications: Hypomobility in any scapular depression muscles.

Scapulothoracic

Inferior Glide

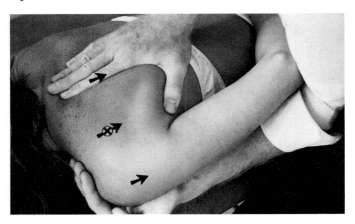

Patient Position: Patient lies prone or is side-lying, with the shoulder girdle in the anatomic position (LPP). (a) In prone, the patient's hand is placed in the small of the back. (b) In side-lying, the patient's upper arm rests on the lateral chest wall.

Therapist Position: (a) With the patient prone, the therapist stands along the side to be mobilized facing the patient. The therapist's cephalic arm cradles the patient's upper extremity. (b) With the patient side-lying, the therapist faces the patient with the therapist's caudal hand resting under the patient's arm.

Stabilization: Provided by the patient's body weight.

Mobilization: With the patient prone or side-lying, the therapist's cephalic hand supports the scapula anteriorly at the coracoid process; the caudal hand grasps under the medial border of the scapula.

Direction of Force: Therapist's hands glide the scapula inferiorly along the thoracic wall.

Indications: Hypomobility in any scapular elevator muscles.

Scapulothoracic

Medial Glide

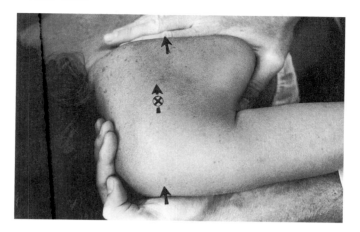

Patient Position: Patient lies prone or is side-lying, with the shoulder girdle in the anatomic position (LPP). (a) In prone, the patient's arm is placed in the small of the back. (b) In side-lying, the patient's upper arm rests on the lateral chest wall.

Therapist Position: (a) With the patient prone, the therapist stands along the side to be mobilized facing the patient. The therapist's cephalic arm cradles the patient's upper extremity. (b) With the patient side-lying, the therapist faces the patient with the therapist's caudal hand resting under the patient's arm.

Stabilization: Provided by the patient's body weight.

Mobilization: With the patient prone or side-lying, the therapist's cephalic hand supports the scapula anteriorly at the coracoid process; the caudal hand grasps under the medial border of the scapula.

Direction of Force: Therapist's hands glide the scapula in a medial direction.

Indications: Hypomobility in any scapular protractor muscles.

Scapulothoracic

Lateral Glide

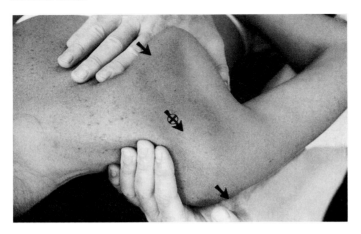

Patient Position: Patient lies prone or is side-lying, with the shoulder girdle in the anatomic position (LPP). (a) In prone, the patient's hand is placed in the small of the back. (b) In side-lying, the patient's upper arm rests on the lateral chest wall.

Therapist Position: (a) With the patient prone, the therapist stands along the side to be mobilized facing the patient. The therapist's cephalic arm cradles the patient's upper extremity. (b) With the patient side-lying, the therapist faces the patient with the therapist's caudal hand resting under the patient's arm.

Stabilization: Provided by the patient's body weight.

Mobilization: With the patient prone or side-lying the therapist's cephalic hand supports the scapula anteriorly at the coracoid process; the caudal hand grasps under the medial border of the scapula.

Direction of Force: Therapist's hands glide the scapula laterally along the thoracic wall.

Indications: Hypomobility in any scapular retractor muscles.

Scapulothoracic

Medial Rotation

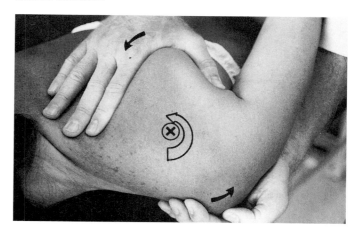

Patient Position: Patient lies prone or is side-lying, with the shoulder girdle in the anatomic position (LPP). In prone, the patient's hand is placed in the small of the back. In side-lying, the patient's upper arm rests on the lateral chest wall.

Therapist Position: (a) With the patient prone, the therapist stands along the side to be mobilized facing the patient. The therapist's cephalic arm cradles the patient's upper extremity. (b) With the patient side-lying, the therapist faces the patient with the therapist's caudal hand resting under the patient's arm.

Stabilization: Provided by the patient's body weight.

Mobilization: With the patient prone or side-lying, the therapist's cephalic hand supports the scapula anteriorly at the coracoid process; the caudal hand grasps under the medial border of the scapula.

Direction of Force: Therapist's hands rotate the scapula medially along the thoracic wall.

Indications: Hypomobility in any scapular lateral rotator muscles.

Scapulothoracic

Lateral Rotation

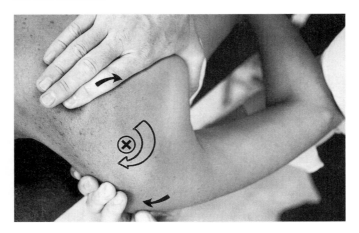

Patient Position: Patient lies prone or is side-lying, with the shoulder girdle in the anatomic position. In prone, the patient's hand is placed in the small of the back. In side-lying, the patient's upper arm rests on the lateral chest wall.

Therapist Position: (a) With the patient prone, the therapist stands along the side to be mobilized facing the patient. The therapist's cephalic arm cradles the patient's upper extremity. (b) With the patient side-lying, the therapist faces the patient with the therapist's caudal hand resting under the patient's arm.

Stabilization: Provided by the patient's body weight.

Mobilization: With the patient prone or side-lying, the therapist's cephalic hand supports the scapula anteriorly at the coracoid process; the caudal hand grasps under the medial border of the scapula.

Direction of Force: Therapist's hands rotate the scapula laterally along the thoracic wall.

Indications: Hypomobility in any scapular medial rotator muscles.

LOWER EXTREMITY

Hip

Flexion Overpressure (with Knee Flexion)

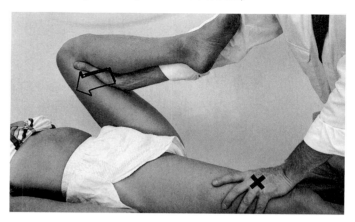

Patient Position: Patient lies supine.

Therapist Position: Therapist stands alongside facing the patient.

Stabilization: Therapist's cephalic hand stabilizes the opposite extremity above the knee.

Mobilization: Therapist's caudal hand supports the lower extremity in the popliteal fossa with the knee flexed.

Direction of Force: Therapist's mobilizing hand flexes the hip to the end of range.

Hip

Flexion Overpressure (with Knee Extension)

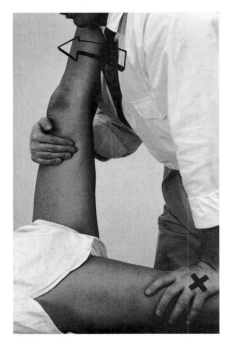

Patient Position: Patient lies supine.

Therapist Position: Therapist stands alongside facing the patient.

Stabilization: Therapist's caudal hand stabilizes the contralateral extremity above the knee.

Mobilization: Therapist positions the patient's distal leg and foot on the therapist's shoulder while maintaining knee extension with the cephalic hand positioned over the anterior caudal femur.

Direction of Force: Therapist's mobilizing hand and trunk flex the hip to the end of range.

Hip

Extension Overpressure

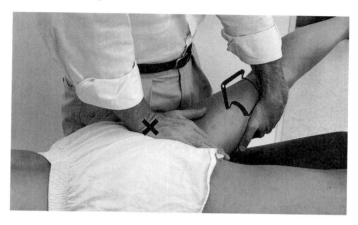

Patient Position: Patient lies prone.

Therapist Position: Therapist stands along the side to be tested.

Stabilization: Therapist's cephalic hand stabilizes the ipsilateral ischial tuberosity in an anterior inferior direction.

Mobilization: Therapist's caudal hand grasps the anterior caudal femur with the knee extended or flexed to 90°.

Direction of Force: Therapist's mobilizing hand extends the hip to the end of range.

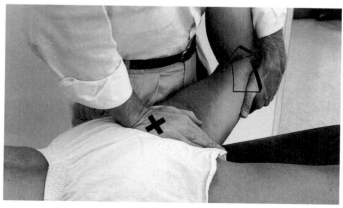

Extension Overpressure with Knee Flexion

Hip

Abduction Overpressure

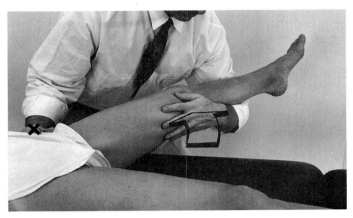

Patient Position: Patient lies supine.

Therapist Position: Therapist stands along the side to be tested.

Stabilization: Therapist's cephalic hand stabilizes the ipsilateral (or contra-lateral) ilium.

Mobilization: Therapist's caudal hand cradles the leg (knee extended) or grasps the medial caudal femur (knee flexed).

Direction of Force: Therapist's mobilizing hand abducts the hip to the end of range.

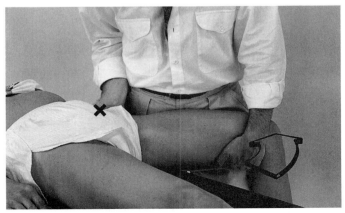

Abduction Overpressure with Knee Flexion

Hip

Adduction Overpressure (Supine)

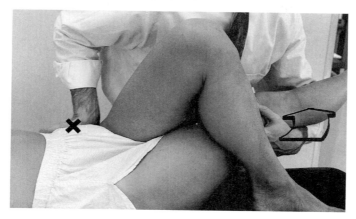

Patient Position: Patient lies supine with the contralateral extremity crossed (figure above) over the extremity to be tested or uncrossed (figure below).

Therapist Position: Therapist stands opposite of the side being tested.

Stabilization: Therapist's cephalic hand stabilizes the ipsilateral or contralateral ilium.

Mobilization: Therapist's caudal hand cradles the extremity above the knee with the knee extended.

Direction of Force: Therapist's mobilizing hand adducts the hip to the end of range.

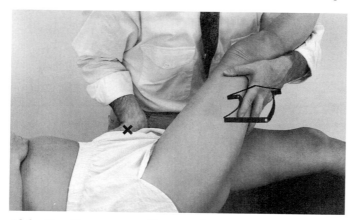

Abduction Overpressure Uncrossed

Hip

Adduction Overpressure (Side-lying)

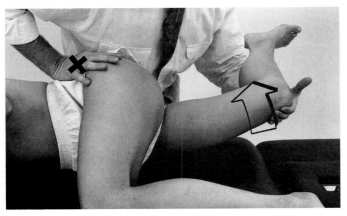

Patient Position: Patient is side-lying with both legs flexed at the hip and knee.

Therapist Position: Therapist stands behind the patient.

Stabilization: Therapist's cephalic hand stabilizes the superior ilium in a caudal direction.

Mobilization: Therapist's caudal hand cradles the inferior leg at the femur maintaining the hip in neutral and the knee flexed.

Direction of Force: Therapist's mobilizing hand adducts the hip to the end of range.

Hip

External Rotation Overpressure (Supine)

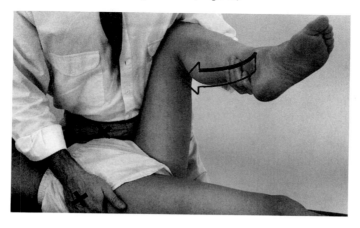

Patient Position: Patient lies supine with the hip and knee flexed to 90°.

Therapist Position: Therapist stands along the side to be tested.

Stabilization: Therapist's cephalic hand stabilizes the contralateral ilium. Therapist's body also provides stabilization.

Mobilization: Therapist's caudal hand grasps the lateral caudal tibia and fibula while simultaneously positioning the patient's knee in (or near) the therapist's axilla.

Direction of Force: Therapist's mobilizing hand and trunk externally rotate the hip to the end of range.

Hip

External Rotation Overpressure (Prone)

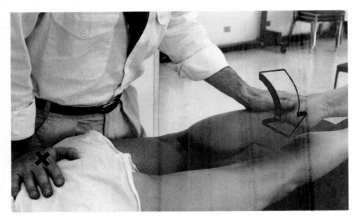

Patient Position: Patient lies prone with the knee flexed to 90°.

Therapist Position: Therapist stands along the side to be tested.

Stabilization: Therapist's cephalic hand stabilizes the ipsilateral ilium.

Mobilization: Therapist's caudal hand grasps the lower leg above the ankle.

Direction of Force: Therapist's mobilizing hand externally rotates the hip to the end of range.

Hip

Internal Rotation Overpressure (Supine)

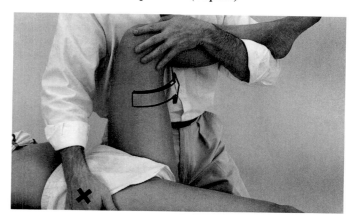

Patient Position: Patient lies supine with the hip and knee flexed to 90°.

Therapist Position: Therapist stands along the side to be tested.

Stabilization: Therapist's cephalic hand stabilizes the opposite ilium. Therapist's body also provides stabilization.

Mobilization: Therapist's caudal hand cradles the lower leg medially supporting it between the forearm and trunk.

Direction of Force: Therapist's mobilizing hand and trunk internally rotate the hip to the end of range.

Hip

Internal Rotation Overpressure (Prone)

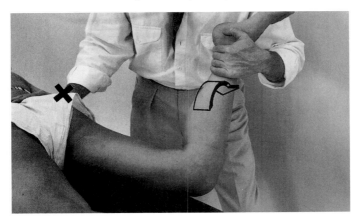

Patient Position: Patient lies prone with the knee flexed to 90°.

Therapist Position: Therapist stands along the side to be tested.

Stabilization: Therapist's cephalic hand stabilizes the ipsilateral ilium.

Mobilization: Therapist's caudal hand grasps the lower leg above the ankle.

Direction of Force: Therapist's mobilizing hand internally rotates the hip to the end of range.

Knee

Flexion Overpressure (Supine)

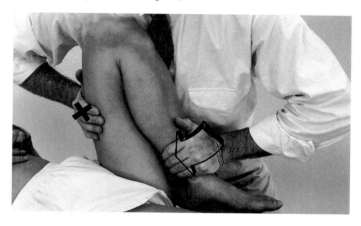

Patient Position: Patient lies supine with the hip in 90° flexion.

Therapist Position: Therapist stands along the side to be tested.

Stabilization: Therapist's cephalic hand grasps the anterior femur. Therapist's body also provides stabilization.

Mobilization: Therapist's caudal hand grasps the lower leg anteriorly above the ankle.

Direction of Force: Therapist's mobilizing hand flexes the knee to the end of range.

Knee

Flexion Overpressure (Prone)

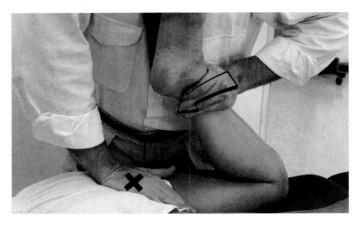

Patient Position: Patient lies prone.

Therapist Position: Therapist stands along the side to be tested.

Stabilization: Therapist's cephalic hand stabilizes over the ischial tuberosity.

Mobilization: Therapist's caudal hand grasps the lower leg above the ankle.

Direction of Force: Therapist's mobilizing hand flexes the knee to the end of range.

Knee

Extension Overpressure

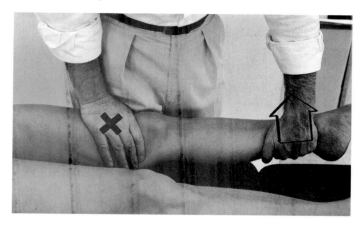

Patient Position: Patient lies supine.

Therapist Position: Therapist stands along the side to be tested.

Stabilization: Therapist's cephalic hand stabilizes the anterior caudal femur above the knee.

Mobilization: Therapist's caudal hand grasps the lower leg posteriorly above the ankle.

Direction of Force: Therapist's mobilizing hand extends the knee to the end of range.

Knee

External Rotation Overpressure

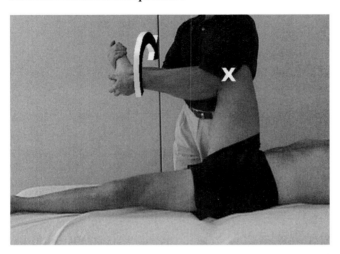

Patient Position: Patient lies supine with the hip and knee flexed to 90°.

Therapist Position: Therapist stands along the side to be tested.

Stabilization: Therapist's cephalic upper arm/elbow holds the lower leg against his/her body.

Mobilization: Therapist's caudal hand grasps the forefoot while his/her cephalic hand grasps the calcaneus.

Direction of Force: Therapist's mobilizing hands externally rotate the tibia to the end of range.

Knee

Internal Rotation Overpressure

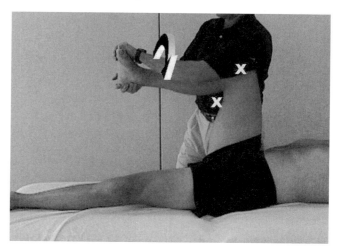

Patient Position: Patient lies supine with the hip and the knee flexed to 90°.

Therapist Position: Therapist stands along the side to be tested.

Stabilization: Therapist's cephalic upper arm/elbow holds the lower leg against his/her body.

Mobilization: Therapist's caudal hand grasps the calcaneus while his/her cephalic hand grasps the forefoot.

Direction of Force: Therapist's mobilizing hands internally rotate the tibia to the end of range.

Ankle/Foot

Dorsiflexion Overpressure

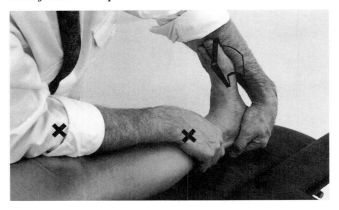

Patient Position: Patient lies supine with (a) hips and knees extended or (b) hips and knees flexed to 90°.

Therapist Position: Therapist stands along the side to be tested.

Stabilization: Therapist's cephalic hand and forearm stabilize the leg and distal tibia and fibula. Therapist's cephalic hand grasps the anterior caudal femur. Therapist's body also provides stabilization.

Mobilization: Maintaining a neutral subtalar position, the therapist's caudal hand grasps the calcaneus placing the anterior forearm along the plantar surface of the patient's foot.

Direction of Force: Therapist's mobilizing hand and forearm dorsiflexes the ankle to the end of range.

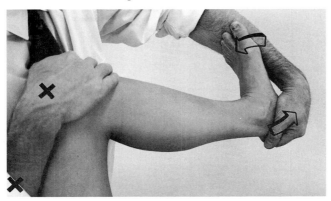

Dorsiflexion Overpressure with Hip and Knee Flexion

Ankle/Foot

Plantar Flexion Overpressure

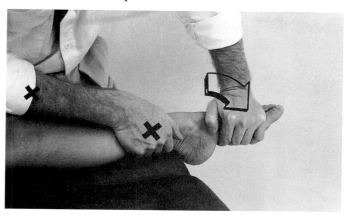

Patient Position: Patient lies supine.

Therapist Position: Therapist stands along the side to be tested.

Stabilization: Therapist's cephalic hand grasps the posterior lower leg above the ankle.

Mobilization: Therapist's caudal hand grasps the dorsal forefoot.

Direction of Force: Therapist's mobilizing hand plantar flexes the ankle to the end of range.

Ankle/Foot

Eversion Overpressure (Subtalar)

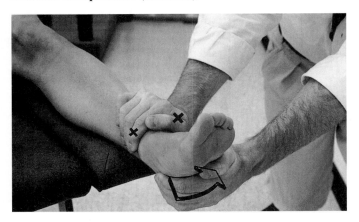

Patient Position: Patient lies supine.

Therapist Position: Therapist stands along the side to be tested.

Stabilization: Therapist's cephalic hand grasps the lateral malleolus.

Mobilization: Therapist's caudal hand grasps the calcaneus.

Direction of Force: Therapist's mobilizing hand everts the ankle to the end of range.

Ankle/Foot

Inversion Overpressure (Subtalar)

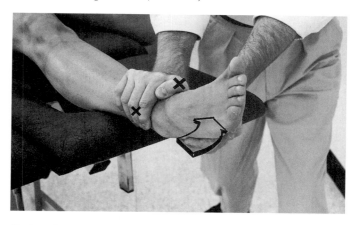

Patient Position: Patient lies supine.

Therapist Position: Therapist stands along the medial side of the patient.

Stabilization: Therapist's cephalic hand grasps the medial malleolus.

Mobilization: Therapist's caudal hand grasps the calcaneus.

Direction of Force: Therapist's mobilizing hand inverts the ankle to the end of range.

Ankle/Foot

Eversion Overpressure (Midtarsal)

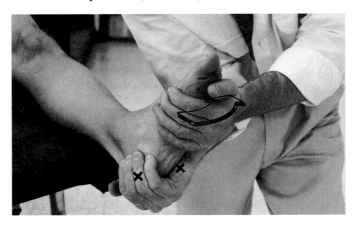

Patient Position: Patient lies supine.

Therapist Position: Therapist stands along the side to be tested.

Stabilization: Therapist's cephalic hand grasps the posterior calcaneus.

Mobilization: Therapist's caudal hand grasps the medial forefoot.

Direction of Force: Therapist's mobilizing hand everts the forefoot to the end of range.

Ankle/Foot

Inversion Overpressure (Midtarsal)

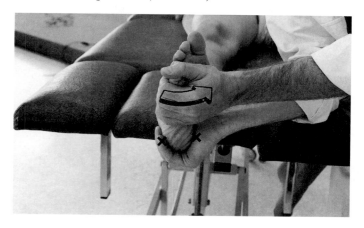

Patient Position: Patient lies supine.

Therapist Position: Therapist stands on the opposite side to be tested.

Stabilization: Therapist's cephalic hand grasps the posterior calcaneus.

Mobilization: Therapist's caudal hand grasps the lateral forefoot.

Direction of Force: Therapist's mobilizing hand inverts the forefoot to the end of range.

Toe

Extension Overpressure

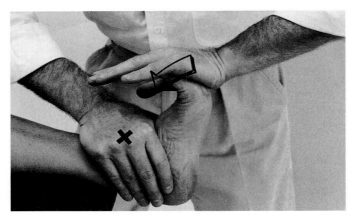

Patient Position: Patient lies supine.

Therapist Position: Therapist stands along the side to be tested.

Stabilization: Therapist's cephalic hand grasps the patient's forefoot.

Mobilization: Therapist's caudal hand grasps the plantar surface of the toes as a group or individually.

Direction of Force: Therapist's mobilizing hand extends the toes to the end of the range.

Toe

Flexion Overpressure

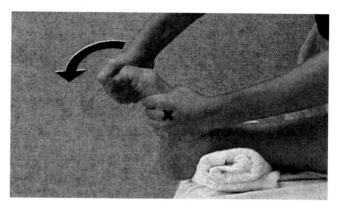

Patient Position: Patient lies supine.

Therapist Position: Therapist stands along the side to be tested.

Stabilization: Therapist's cephalic hand grasps the patient's forefoot.

Mobilization: Therapist's caudal hand grasps the dorsal surface of the toes as a group or individually.

Direction of Force: Therapist's mobilizing hand flexes the toes to the end of the range.

Hip

Long Axis Traction

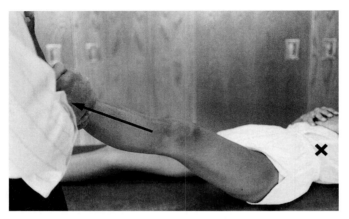

Patient Position: Patient lies supine with the hip in 30° flexion, 30° abduction, and slight external rotation (LPP). The knee can be flexed or extended.

Therapist Position: Therapist stands alongside the patient's leg to be mobilized, facing the patient, with the foot or knee stabilized against the therapist's abdomen.

Stabilization: Patient's body weight provides stabilization.

Mobilization: Therapist grasps above the ankle with both hands around the tibia and fibula, one hand anterior and the other hand posterior.

Direction of Force: Therapist distracts the hip joint through the long axis of the femur.

Indications: To decrease superior femoral contact surface area and inferior capsular hypomobility.

Hip

Long Axis Compression

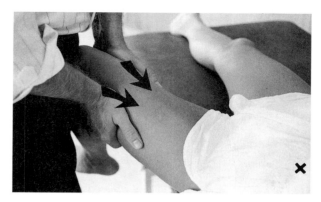

Patient Position: Patient lies supine with the hip in 30° flexion, 30° abduction, and slight external rotation (LPP). The knee can be flexed or extended.

Therapist Position: Therapist stands alongside the patient's leg to be mobilized, facing the patient, with the foot or knee stabilized against the therapist's abdomen.

Stabilization: Patient's body weight provides stabilization.

Mobilization: Therapist grasps both sides of the knee at the distal femur (knee flexed) or the distal tibia and fibula (knee extended).

Direction of Force: Therapist compresses the hip joint through the long axis of the femur.

Indication: Provocation findings with superior femoral contact area changes.[1]

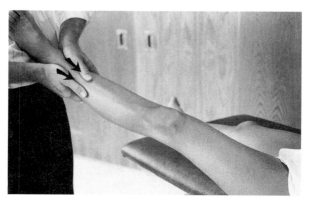

Long Axis Compression with Knee Extension

Hip

Lateral Distraction

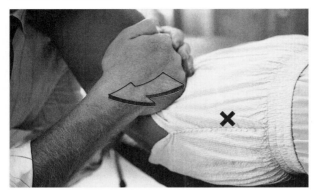

Patient Position: Patient lies supine with the hip in 30° of flexion, 30° of abduction, and slight external rotation (LPP) with the hip joint off the edge of the table.

Therapist Position: Therapist stands alongside the leg to be mobilized facing the patient. Therapist places the patient's lower extremity over the therapist's medial shoulder maintaining the LPP.

Stabilization: Patient's body weight provides stabilization.

Mobilization: Therapist grasps the proximal anterior and medial femur with both hands.

Direction of Force: Therapist distracts the hip in an anterior, lateral, and inferior direction.

Indication: Any capsular hypomobility.

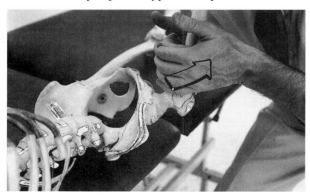

Skeletal Hip Lateral Distraction

Hip

Compression

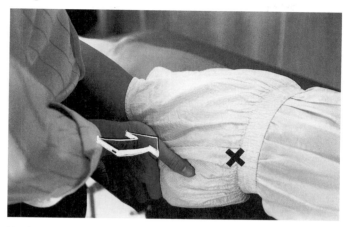

Patient Position: Patient lies supine with the hip in 30° of flexion, 30° of abduction, and slight external rotation (LPP) with the hip joint off the edge of the table.

Therapist Position: Therapist stands alongside the leg to be mobilized facing the patient. Therapist holds the patient's lower extremity under the knee maintaining the LPP with the medial hand.

Stabilization: Patient's body weight provides stabilization.

Mobilization: Therapist places the cephalic hand over the greater trochanter.

Direction of Force: Therapist compresses the hip in a posterior, medial, and superior direction.

Indication: Provocation findings with arthritis.[1]

Hip

Anterior Glide

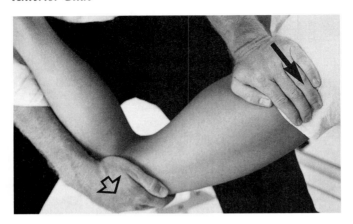

Patient Position: Patient lies prone with the anterior superior iliac spine (ASIS) firmly supported (towel, wedge, etc.) and the hip in 30° of flexion, 30° abduction, and slight external rotation (LPP). The knee is flexed with the femur off the side of the table.

Therapist Position: Therapist stands inside the patient's lower extremity supporting the flexed knee with the caudal hand.

Stabilization: Table and towel/wedge provide stabilization.

Mobilization: Therapist places the cephalic hand over the proximal posterior and lateral femur. Piccolo distraction prior to mobilization is provided by the therapist's cephalic leg moving the femur laterally.

Direction of Force: Therapist glides the femur in an anterior and medial direction.

Indications: Extension hypomobility and external rotation hypomobility.

Hip

Posterior Glide

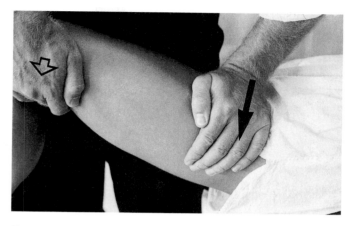

Patient Position: Patient lies supine with the hip in 30° of flexion, 30° of abduction, and slight external rotation (LPP). The knee is flexed with the femur off the side of the table.

Therapist Position: Therapist stands inside the lower extremity supporting the distal femur with the caudal hand.

Stabilization: Patient's body weight and table provide stabilization.

Mobilization: Therapist places the cephalic hand over the proximal anterior and medial femur. Piccolo distraction prior to mobilization is provided by the therapist's cephalic leg moving the femur laterally.

Direction of Force: Therapist glides the femur in a posterior and lateral direction.

Indications: Flexion hypomobility and internal rotation hypomobility.

Hip

External Rotation

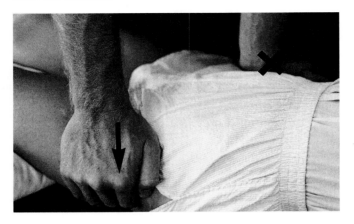

Patient Position: Patient lies supine with the lower extremity in a neutral position and a pillow under both knees.

Therapist Position: Therapist stands opposite the side to be mobilized.

Stabilization: Therapist stabilizes the opposite anterior superior iliac spine (ASIS).

Mobilization: Therapist grasps the greater trochanter on the side to be mobilized with a lumbrical grip.

Direction of Force: Therapist moves the greater trochanter in a posterior direction externally rotating the lower extremity.

Indication: External rotation hypomobility.

Hip

Internal Rotation

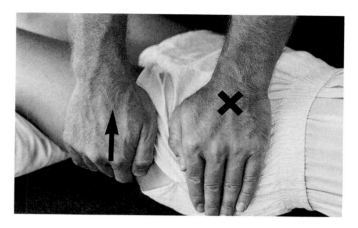

Patient Position: Patient lies supine with the lower extremity in a neutral position and a pillow under both knees.

Therapist Position: Therapist stands opposite the side to be mobilized.

Stabilization: Therapist stabilizes the anterior superior iliac spine (ASIS) on the side to be mobilized.

Mobilization: Therapist grasps the greater trochanter with a lumbrical grip on the side to be mobilized.

Direction of Force: Therapist moves the greater trochanter in an anterior direction internally rotating the lower extremity.

Indication: Internal rotation hypomobility.

Hip

Fabere's/Patrick's Test

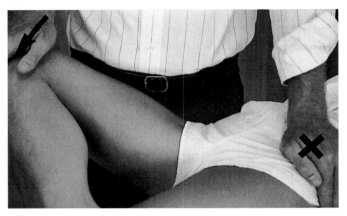

This is a test for hip (or sacroiliac) pathology.

Patient Position: Patient lies supine with the leg in flexion, abduction, and external rotation resting the ankle on the opposite leg above the knee.

Therapist Position: Therapist stands alongside the leg to be tested.

Stabilization: Therapist's cephalic hand is placed over the anterior superior iliac spine (ASIS) on the opposite side.

Mobilization: Therapist's caudal hand grasps the distal medial femur.

Direction of Force: Therapist lowers the femur into the combined movements of extension, abduction, and external rotation.

Indications: Provocation findings are suggestive of hip (or sacroiliac) pathology.

Hip

Scour/Quadrant Test

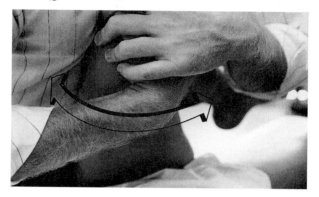

Patient Position: Patient lies supine with the hip to be tested in full flexion and adduction. The knee is relaxed in flexion.

Therapist Position: Therapist can stand on either side of the patient.

Stabilization: Patient's body weight provides stabilization.

Mobilization: Therapist grasps around the distal femur without compressing the patella/femoral joint.

Direction of Force: Therapist applies a slight posterior force along the shaft of the femur maintaining the adducted position. The hip is then slowly extended to a position of about 90° of flexion. This movement is repeated several times.

Indication: An abnormality in this movement associated with arthritis maybe felt as a small hump or a defect along the arc of motion which may reproduce symptoms.

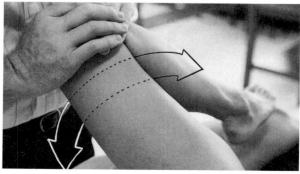

Scour/Quadrant Test's Arc of Motion

Femoral/Tibial

Distraction (Sitting)

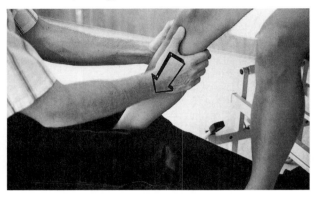

Patient Position: Patient sits on the table with the knee flexed 30° (LPP) with a small towel placed under the distal femur.

Therapist Position: Therapist sits facing the patient with the patient's lower leg supported between the knees of the therapist.

Stabilization: The distal femur is stabilized by a towel and the table.

Mobilization: Therapist grasps the proximal tibia with both hands palpating the joint line with the thumbs.

Direction of Force: The knee is distracted by pulling the tibia in a caudal direction by both the legs and hands of the therapist.

Indication: Any capsular hypomobility.

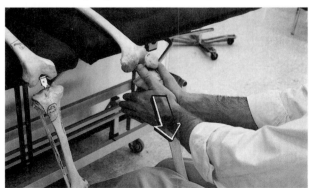

Skeletal Femoral/Tibial Distraction

Femoral/Tibial

Distraction (Prone)

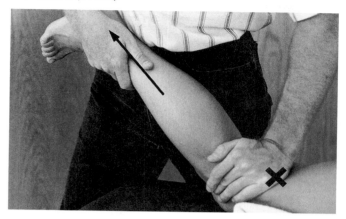

Patient Position: Patient lies prone with the leg in 30° of flexion (LPP) with a small towel placed under the distal anterior femur.

Therapist Position: Therapist stands alongside the patient's leg.

Stabilization: Therapist's cephalic hand stabilizes the distal posterior surface of the femur while palpating the joint line.

Mobilization: Therapist's caudal hand grasps the distal tibia with the lower leg supported by the therapist's body.

Direction of Force: Therapist pulls the tibia in a caudal direction distracting the knee.

Indication: Any capsular hypomobility.

Femoral/Tibial

Compression (Sitting)

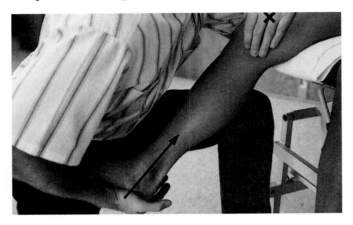

Patient Position: Patient sits on the table with the knee flexed to 30° (LPP).

Therapist Position: Therapist sits or kneels facing the patient's leg.

Stabilization: Therapist's cephalic hand provides stabilization to the anterior distal surface of the femur while palpating the joint line.

Mobilization: Therapist's caudal hand grasps the foot/ankle with the lower leg supported by part of the therapist's body.

Direction of Force: Therapist pushes the tibia in an anterior and cephalic direction compressing the knee.

Indication: Provocation with arthritis.[1]

Femoral/Tibial

Compression (Prone)

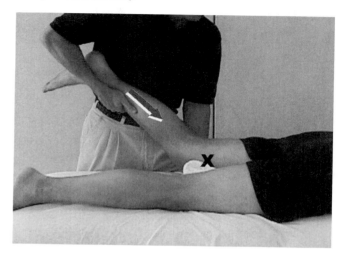

Patient Position: Patient lies prone with the knee flexed to 30° (LPP).

Therapist Position: Therapist stands alongside the patient's leg.

Stabilization: The table and a towel placed cephalic to the patella provide stabilization of the distal femur. Therapist's cephalic hand stabilizes the distal femur while palpating the joint line.

Mobilization: Therapist's caudal hand grasps the lower leg.

Direction of Force: Therapist pushes the tibia in an anterior and cephalic direction compressing the knee.

Indication: Provocation findings with arthritis.[1]

Femoral/Tibial

Anterior Glide (Prone)

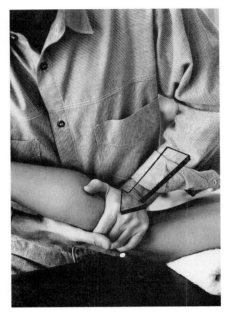

Patient Position: Patient lies prone or sits with the knee flexed to 30° (LPP) with a small towel placed under the distal femur.

Therapist Position: Therapist stands or kneels alongside the patient's leg.

Stabilization: Stabilization is provided by the towel and/or table.

Mobilization: Therapist supports the patient's anterior lower leg with the caudal arm while palpating the anterior joint line. The cephalic hand is placed over the posterior aspect of the proximal tibia (top figure).

Direction of Force: Therapist glides the tibia in an anterior direction.

Indication: Extension hypomobility.

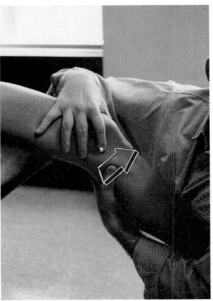

Anterior Glide (Sitting)

Femoral/Tibial

Posterior Glide (Sitting)

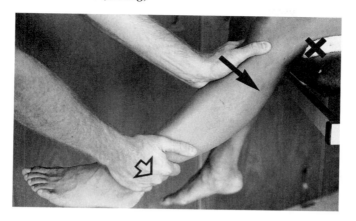

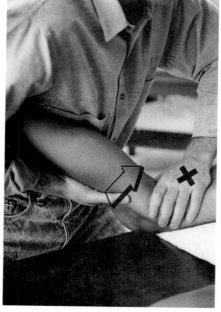

Patient Position: Patient sits or lies prone with the knee flexed to 30° (LPP).

Therapist Position: Therapist stands facing the patient's leg.

Stabilization: Stabilization is provided by the towel and table.

Mobilization: Therapist grasps the distal lower leg with one hand and places the other hand over the anterior aspect of the proximal tibia (top figure).

Direction of Force: Therapist glides the tibia in a posterior direction.

Indication: Flexion hypomobility.

Posterior Glide (Prone)

Femoral/Tibial

Medial/Lateral Rotation

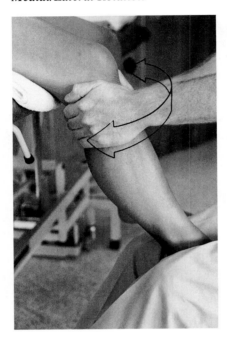

Patient Position: Patient sits on the table with the knee flexed to 30° (LPP).

Therapist Position: Therapist sits facing the patient with the patient's lower leg supported between the knee's of the therapist.

Stabilization: The distal femur is stabilized by a towel and the table.

Mobilization: Therapist grasps the proximal tibia with both hands while palpating the joint line with the thumbs.

Direction of Force: Rotation is produced by pulling with one hand and pushing with the other.

Indications: Flexion hypomobility (medial); extension hypomobility (lateral).

NOTE: It is important to (a) attempt to produce rotation of the tibia and not just two independent glides; (b) allow the lower leg to rotate; and (c) have the therapist positioned more toward the side of the direction of the rotation to be produced.

Femoral/Tibial

Medial Tilt/Valgus Stress Test

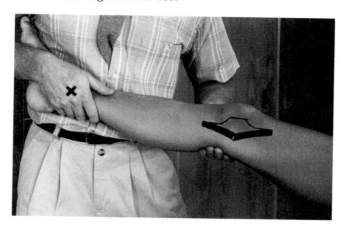

Patient Position: Patient lies supine.

Therapist Position: Therapist stands facing the lateral side of the leg to be tested.

Stabilization: Therapist supports the patient's distal lower leg with the caudal hand and trunk.

Mobilization: Therapist's cephalic hand supports the popliteal fossa with the fingers maintaining a few degrees of flexion of the knee (figure above) and in 20 to 30° of flexion. The heel of the hand is then placed at the lateral joint line.

Direction of Force: Therapist's cephalic hand pushes in a medial direction while the caudal hand and trunk pull in a lateral direction.

Indications: Extension hypomobility; medial capsule and collateral ligament involvement with stress testing.

Femoral/Tibial

Lateral Tilt/Varus Stress Test

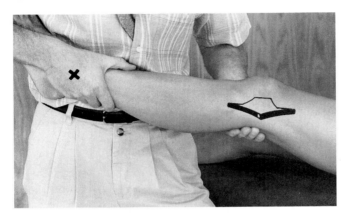

Patient Position: Patient lies supine.

Therapist Position: Therapist stands on the inside of the leg to be tested facing laterally.

Stabilization: Therapist supports the patient's distal lower leg with the caudal hand and trunk.

Mobilization: Therapist's cephalic hand supports the popliteal fossa with the fingers maintaining a few degrees of flexion of the knee (figure above) and in 20 to 30° of flexion. The heel of the hand is then placed at the medial joint line.

Direction of Force: Therapist's cephalic hand pushes in a lateral direction while the caudal hand and trunk pull in a medial direction.

Indications: Flexion hypomobility; lateral capsule and collateral ligament involvement with stress testing.

Patella/Femoral

Distraction

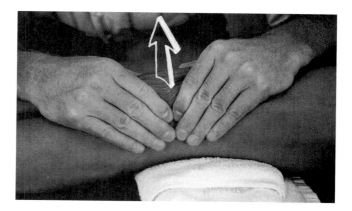

Patient Position: Patient lies supine with the knee in extension (LPP).

Therapist Position: Therapist stands alongside the patient's knee.

Stabilization: The weight of the patient's leg provides stabilization.

Mobilization: Therapist's hands (fingers and thumbs) grasp around the borders of the patella.

Direction of Force: Therapist's mobilizing hands gently lift up on the patella distracting the patella/femoral joint.

Indication: Any capsular hypomobility.

Patella/Femoral

Compression

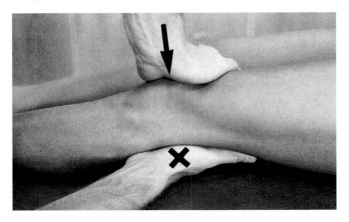

Patient Position: Patient lies supine with the knee in extension (LPP).

Therapist Position: Therapist stands alongside the patient's knee.

Stabilization: The table and the therapist's hand under the popliteal region provide stabilization.

Mobilization: Therapist's other hand is placed over the entire anterior surface of the patella.

Direction of Force: Therapist's mobilizing hand gently pushes down on the patella compressing the patella/femoral joint.

Indication: Provocation findings with arthritis.[1]

It is important to apply pressure slowly so gliding movements are not produced.

Patella/Femoral

Cephalic Glide

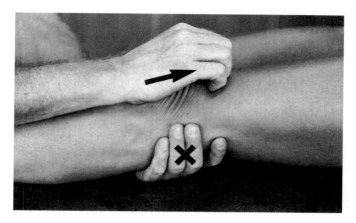

Patient Position: Patient lies supine with the knee in extension (LPP).

Therapist Position: Therapist stands opposite the leg to be mobilized facing the patient's head.

Stabilization: Patient's body weight provides stabilization. Therapist's one hand grasps under the popliteal region.

Mobilization: Therapist's other hand (heel) grasps the inferior border of the patella with the forearm parallel to the patient's lower leg.

Direction of Force: Therapist's mobilizing hand glides the patella superiorly.

Indication: Extension hypomobility.

Patella/Femoral

Caudal Glide

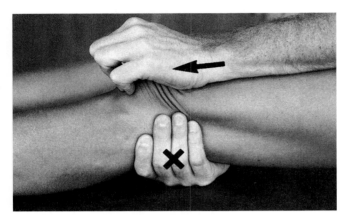

Patient Position: Patient lies supine with the knee in extension (LPP).

Therapist Position: Therapist stands alongside the patient's knee.

Stabilization: Patient's body weight provides stabilization. Therapist's one hand grasps under the popliteal region.

Mobilization: Therapist's other hand (heel) grasps the cephalic border of the patella with the forearm parallel to the patient's thigh.

Direction of Force: Therapist's mobilizing hand glides the patella in a caudal direction.

Indication: Flexion hypomobility.

Patella/Femoral

Medial Glide

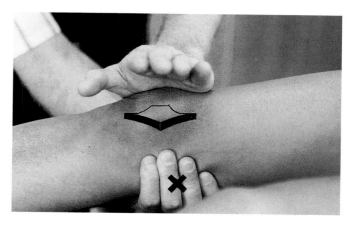

Patient Position: Patient lies supine with the knee in extension (LPP).

Therapist Position: Therapist stands alongside the patient's knee.

Stabilization: Therapist's one hand grasps under the popliteal region and supports the medial side of the knee.

Mobilization: Therapist's other hand (heel) is placed over the lateral border of the patella with the forearm parallel to the leg.

Direction of Force: Therapist glides the patella in a medial direction.

Indications: Extension hypomobility and flexion hypomobility.

Patella/Femoral

Lateral Glide/Apprehension Test

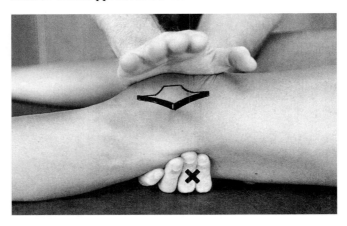

Patient Position: Patient lies supine with the knee in extension (LPP).

Therapist Position: Therapist stands alongside the patient's knee.

Stabilization: Therapist's one hand grasps under the popliteal region and supports the lateral side of the knee.

Mobilization: Therapist's other hand (heel) is placed over the medial border of the patella with the forearm parallel to the leg.

Direction of Force: Therapist glides the patella in a lateral direction.

Indications: Extension hypomobility and flexion hypomobility; provocation findings with subluxation/dislocation hypermobility.

Knee

Apley's Distraction

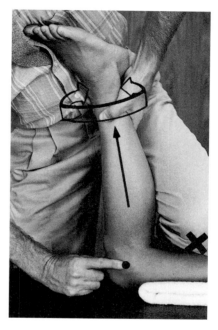

This test is used to distinguish between meniscal and ligamentous problems at the knee.

Patient Position: Patient lies prone with the knee flexed to 90° with a towel placed under the distal anterior femur.

Therapist Position: Therapist stands alongside the patient's knee.

Stabilization: Stabilization provided by the therapist's lower leg over the patient's distal posterior femur.

Mobilization: Therapist grasps the patient's lower leg proximal to the ankle with the cephalic hand. The caudal hand palpates the medial and lateral joint lines.

Direction of Force: Therapist distracts the tibia through the long axis of the bone while producing internal and external rotation of the lower leg.

Indication: Provocation of pain is suggestive of ligamentous damage. If the meniscus alone is torn, the test should not be painful.

Knee

Apley's Compression

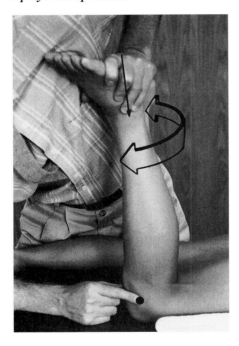

This tests the integrity of the menisci.

Patient Position: Patient lies prone with the knee flexed to 90° with a small towel placed under the distal anterior femur.

Therapist Position: Therapist stands alongside the patient's knee.

Stabilization: Stabilization provided by the table and towel.

Mobilization: Therapist's cephalic hand grasps the plantar aspect of the patient's foot/ankle. The caudal hand palpates the medial and lateral joint lines.

Direction of Force: Therapist applies a compressive force through the long axis of the tibia while producing internal and external rotation of the leg.

Indication: Provocation of pain on either the medial or lateral joint line is suggestive of a meniscal lesion. A click or snap may occur.

Knee

Lachman's Test

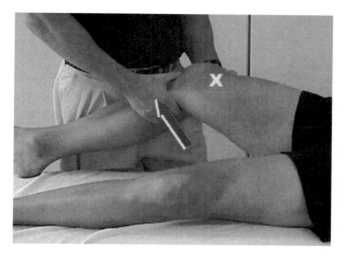

Patient Position: Patient lies supine with the knee flexed approximately 30°.

Therapist Position: Therapist stands facing the patient alongside the knee.

Stabilization: Patient's body weight provides stabilization. Therapist's cephalic hand is placed over the anterior distal femur while palpating the joint lines.

Mobilization: Therapist's caudal arm supports under the patient's lower leg with the hand placed at the proximal posterior tibia.

Direction of Force: Therapist pulls the lower leg upward gliding the tibia in an anterior direction.

Indication: This test assesses anterior instability at the knee, and more specifically, the anterior cruciate ligament.

Knee

Anterior Drawer Test

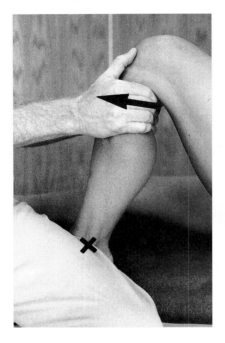

Patient Position: Patient lies supine with the knee flexed to 90° and the foot flat on the table and facing straight ahead (figure). The foot may also be (a) externally rotated 15° or (b) internally rotated 30°.

Therapist Position: Therapist is positioned at the edge of the table, sitting over the patient's foot.

Stabilization: Stabilization is provided by the therapist's weight on the patient's foot and the patient's body weight.

Mobilization: Therapist places the fingers of both hands around the posterior aspect of the proximal tibia with both thumbs placed over the joint lines.

Direction of Force: Therapist pulls the tibia forward on the femur in an anterior direction.

Indications: If the tibia slides forward under the femur (positive drawer), it may suggest a tear of the anterior cruciate ligament. A few degrees of translation are normal if equal to the contralateral side. With external rotation, additional structures including the medial collateral ligament, posteromedial capsule, and posterior oblique ligament may be involved. With internal rotation, additional structures including the lateral collateral ligament, posterolateral capsule, arcuate-popliteus complex, posterior cruciate ligament, and iliotibial band may be involved.[2]

The Lachman test is considered the better examination technique for testing the integrity of the anterior cruciate ligament because of anatomic and practical limitations (90° flexion) to performing an anterior drawer test.[3]

Knee

Posterior Drawer Test

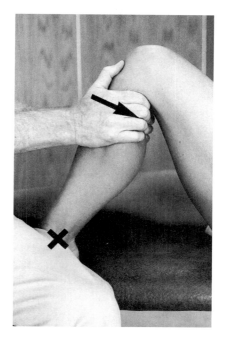

Patient Position: Patient lies supine with the knee flexed to 90° and the foot flat on the table and facing straight ahead (figure). The foot may also be (a) slightly externally rotated or (b) slightly internally rotated.

Therapist Position: Therapist is positioned at the edge of the table sitting over the patient's foot.

Stabilization: Stabilization is provided by the therapist's weight on the patient's foot and the patient's body weight.

Mobilization: Therapist places the heel of both hands over the anterior aspect of the proximal tibia with both thumbs placed over the joint lines.

Direction of Force: Therapist pushes the tibia backward on the femur in a posterior direction.

Indications: If the tibia slides backward on the femur (positive drawer) it may suggest a tear of the posterior cruciate ligament. A few degrees of translation are normal if equal to the contralateral side. With external rotation, additional structures, including the lateral collateral ligament, posterolateral capsule, arcuate popliteal complex, anterior cruciate ligament, and biceps femoris tendon, may be involved. With internal rotation, additional structures, including the medial collateral ligament, posteromedial capsule, posterior oblique ligament, anterior cruciate ligament, and semimembranosus muscle, may be involved.[2]

Knee

McMurray Test (Technique Modified from McMurray's Original Test)[4]

Patient Position: Patient lies supine.

Therapist Position: Therapist stands on the involved side facing the patient's knee.

Test Procedure for Medial Meniscus: Therapist fully flexes the patient's knee. The caudal hand grasps the ankle or distal lower leg and the heel of the cephalic hand is placed over the lateral joint line. The therapist then applies a valgus stress with the cephalic hand and externally rotates the lower leg with the caudal hand. While maintaining both of these forces the knee is slowly lowered down into full extension (figure top of page 183).

Indication: If this technique produces an audible or palpable click within the joint there is a probable tear in the posterior aspect of the medial meniscus.

Test Procedure for Lateral Meniscus: Therapist fully flexes the patient's knee. The caudal hand grasps the ankle or distal lower leg and the heel of the cephalic hand is placed over the medial joint line. The therapist then applies a varus stress with the cephalic hand and internally rotates the lower leg with the caudal hand. While maintaining both of these forces the knee is slowly lowered down into full extension (figure bottom of page 183).

Indication: If this technique produces an audible or palpable click within the joint there is a probable tear in the lateral meniscus.

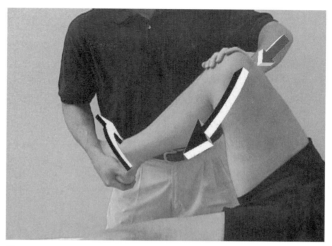

Test Procedure for Medial Meniscus

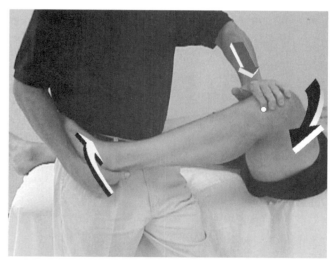

Test Procedure for Lateral Meniscus

Proximal Tibiofibular

Anterior Glide (Prone)

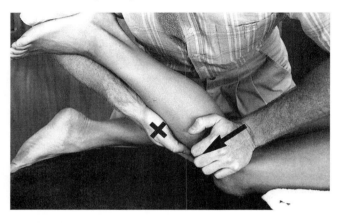

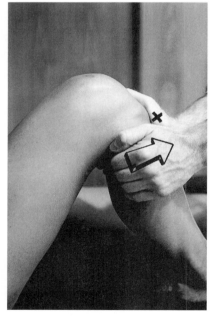

Patient Position: Patient lies prone or sits with the knee midway between flexion and extension and the ankle in 10° of plantar flexion (LPP).

Therapist Position: Therapist stands opposite the patient's lower extremity to be mobilized.

Stabilization: The caudal hand grasps the proximal anterior tibia.

Mobilization: The heel of the cephalic hand grasps the posterior fibular head.

Direction of Force: Therapist glides the fibula on the tibia in an anterior lateral direction.

Indication: Plantar flexion hypomobility.

Anterior Glide (Sitting)

Proximal Tibiofibular

Posterior Glide

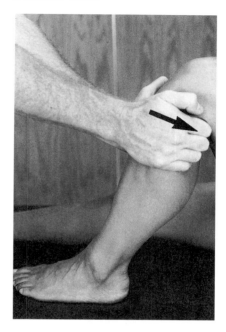

Patient Position: Patient lies supine with the knee midway between flexion and extension and the ankle in 10° of plantar flexion (LPP) with the foot resting on the table.

Therapist Position: Therapist faces the patient's lower extremity to be mobilized.

Stabilization: The medial hand grasps around the proximal posterior portion of the tibia.

Mobilization: The heel of the lateral hand is placed over the anterior portion of the fibular head.

Direction of Force: Therapist glides the fibula on the tibia in a posterior medial direction.

Indication: Dorsiflexion hypomobility.

Proximal Tibiofibular

Cephalic Glide

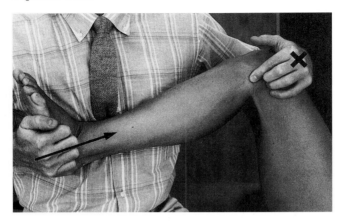

Patient Position: Patient lies supine with the knee midway between flexion and extension and the ankle in 10° of plantar flexion (LPP).

Therapist Position: Therapist stands inside the patient's leg to be mobilized facing laterally.

Stabilization: Therapist's body and cephalic arm are placed over the distal anterior femur while palpating the fibular head.

Mobilization: Therapist's caudal hand grasps the lateral sole of the patient's foot.

Direction of Force: Therapist glides the fibula in a cephalic direction first by dorsiflexing and everting the foot/ankle and second by continuing to push the foot in a cephalic direction.

Indications: Dorsiflexion hypomobility and eversion hypomobility.

Proximal Tibiofibular

Caudal Glide

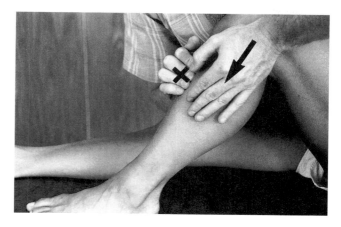

Patient Position: Patient lies supine with the knee midway between flexion and extension and the ankle in 10° of plantar flexion (LPP) with the foot resting on the table.

Therapist Position: Therapist stands alongside the patient's leg.

Stabilization: Therapist's one hand grasps the proximal tibia maintaining it in a cephalic direction.

Mobilization: Therapist grasps the fibular head with the heel of the other hand.

Direction of Force: Therapist glides the fibula on the tibia in a caudal direction.

Indications: Plantar flexion hypomobility and inversion hypomobility.

Distal Tibiofibular

Compression

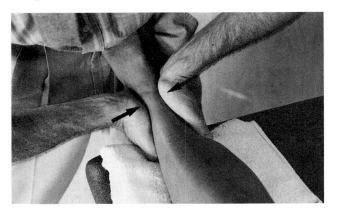

Patient Position: Patient lies supine with the ankle over the edge of the table in 10° of plantar flexion (LPP).

Therapist Position: Therapist stands facing the plantar aspect of the patient's foot.

Stabilization: Patient's foot is stabilized against the therapist's abdomen.

Mobilization: The heel of both hands are placed directly over the malleoli and the forearms are aligned parallel with the floor.

Direction of Force: Therapist slowly pushes both hands together compressing the distal tibiofibular joint.

Indication: Provocation findings with arthritis[1] and syndesmosis rupture.

Distal Tibiofibular

Anterior Glide (Supine)

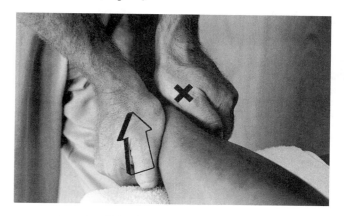

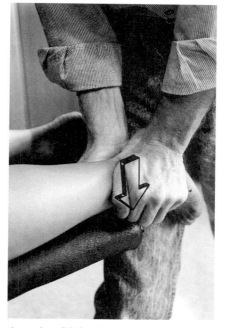

Anterior Glide (Prone)

Patient Position: Patient lies supine with the ankle over the edge of the table in 10° of plantar flexion (LPP).

Therapist Position: Therapist stands facing the plantar aspect of the patient's foot.

Stabilization: The patient's foot rests on the anterior thigh of the therapist. The therapist places the heel of the medial hand over the anterior portion of the medial malleolus.

Mobilization: Therapist's lateral hand grasps the posterior aspect of the lateral malleolus with the fingers.

Direction of Force: Therapist glides the lateral malleolus in an anterior direction.

Indication: Dorsiflexion hypomobility.

Distal Tibiofibular

Posterior Glide

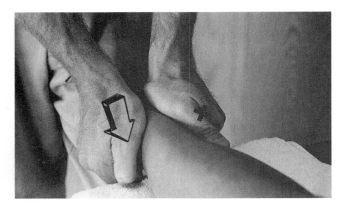

Patient Position: Patient lies supine with the ankle over the edge of the table in 10° of plantar flexion (LPP).

Therapist Position: Therapist stands facing the plantar aspect of the patient's foot.

Stabilization: The patient's foot rests on the anterior thigh of the therapist. The therapist places the fingers of the medial hand under the posterior portion of the medial malleolus.

Mobilization: Therapist places the heel of the lateral hand over the anterior portion of the lateral malleolus.

Direction of Force: Therapist glides the lateral malleolus in a posterior direction.

Indication: Plantar flexion hypomobility.

Talocrural

Distraction

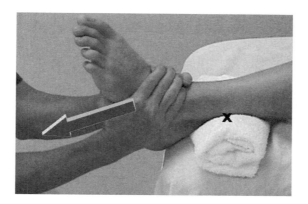

Patient Position: Patient lies supine with slight knee flexion and the ankle over the edge of the table in 10° of plantar flexion and midway betweeen supination and pronation (LPP).

Therapist Position: Therapist stands facing the plantar aspect of the patient's foot.

Stabilization: Patient's body weight provides stabilization.

Mobilization: One of the therapist's hands grasps the patient's forefoot on the dorsal surface placing the fourth or fifth fingers over the talus and the thumb on the plantar surface. The opposite hand is placed over the other with the thumb in a similar position.

Direction of Force: Therapist distracts the talus in a caudal direction.

Indication: Any capsular hypomobility.

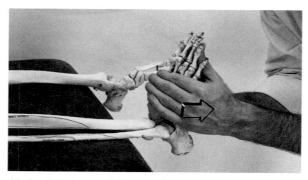

Skeletal Talocrural Distraction

Talocrural

Compression

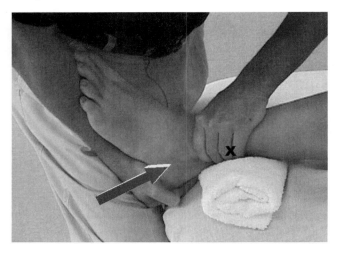

Patient Position: Patient lies supine with slight knee flexion and the ankle over the edge of the table in 10° of plantar flexion and midway betweeen supination and pronation (LPP).

Therapist Position: Therapist stands facing the foot.

Stabilization: Therapist's cephalic hand grasps the distal tibia and fibula anteriorly.

Mobilization: Therapist's caudal hand is placed with the palm covering the plantar aspect of the calcaneus and the forearm supporting the patient's forefoot.

Direction of Force: Therapist compresses the talocrural joint through the calcaneus in a cephalic direction.

Indication: Provocation findings with arthritis.[1]

This technique also compresses the subtalar joint.

Talocrural

Anterior Glide (Supine)/Ligament Stress Test (Anterior Drawer)

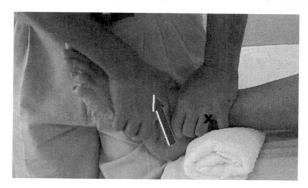

Patient Position: Patient lies supine with ankle over the edge of the table in 10° of plantar flexion and midway betweeen supination and pronation (LPP).

Therapist Position: Therapist stands facing the foot.

Stabilization: Therapist's cephalic hand grasps the distal tibia and fibula anteriorly.

Mobilization: Therapist's caudal hand grasps the anterior talus with a pinch grip between the index finger and thumb while the remaining fingers support the plantar aspect of the patient's foot (figure above). Therapist's caudal hand grasps the posterior talus with a pinch grip between the finger and thumb (figure below).

Direction of Force: Therapist glides the talus in an anterior and a slightly caudal direction.

Indications: Plantar flexion hypomobility; lateral collateral ligament involvement with stress testing.

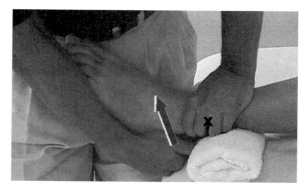

Talocrural

Anterior Glide (Prone)/Ligament Stress Test (Anterior Drawer)

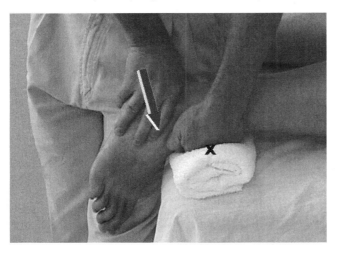

Patient Position: Patient lies prone with the ankle over the edge of the table in 10° of plantar flexion and midway betweeen supination and pronation (LPP).

Therapist Position: Therapist stands facing the foot.

Stabilization: Therapist's cephalic hand grasps the anterior surface of the distal tibia and fibula while supporting the patient's forefoot on the therapist's thigh.

Mobilization: Therapist's caudal hand grasps the posterior talus between the thumb and index finger.

Direction of Force: Therapist glides the talus in an anterior and slightly caudal direction.

Indications: Plantar flexion hypomobility; lateral collateral ligament involvement with stress testing.

Talocrural

Posterior Glide

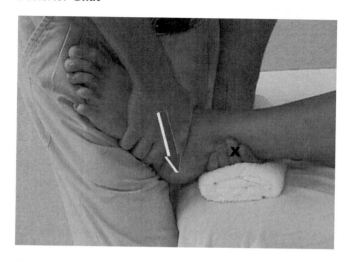

Patient Position: Patient lies supine with the ankle over the edge of the table in 10° of plantar flexion and midway betweeen supination and pronation (LPP).

Therapist Position: Therapist stands facing the foot.

Stabilization: Therapist's cephalic hand grasps the distal tibia and fibula posteriorly.

Mobilization: Therapist's caudal hand grasps the anterior talus between the index finger and thumb while the remaining fingers support the plantar aspect of the patient's foot.

Direction of Force: Therapist glides the talus in a posterior and slightly cephalic direction.

Indications: Dorsiflexion hypomobility.

Subtalar

Distraction (Supine)

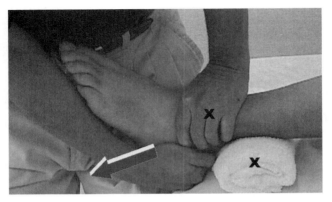

Patient Position: Patient lies supine with the knee slightly flexed and the ankle over the edge of the table midway between supination and pronation (LPP).

Therapist Position: Therapist stands facing the foot.

Stabilization: Therapist's cephalic hand grasps the distal leg and talus on the medial and lateral sides.

Mobilization: Therapist's caudal hand grasps the calcaneus.

Direction of Force: Therapist distracts the calcaneus in a caudal and posterior direction perpendicular to the plane of the calcaneus.

Indication: Any capsular hypomobility.

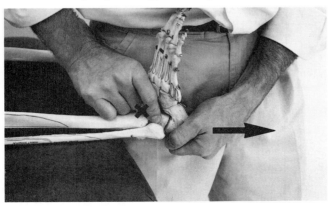

Skeletal Subtalar Distraction

Subtalar

Distraction (Prone)

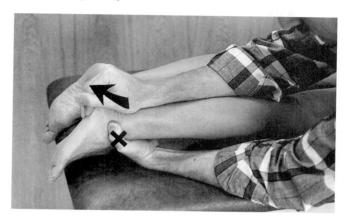

Patient Position: Patient lies prone with slight knee flexion and slight plantar flexion midway between supination and pronation (LPP).

Therapist Position: Therapist stands facing the foot.

Stabilization: Therapist grasps the ventral aspect of the distal leg and talus.

Mobilization: Therapist's mobilization hand grasps the calcaneus with the heel of the hand. Therapist's forearm rests on the patient's calf.

Direction of Force: Therapist distracts the calcaneus in a caudal and posterior direction.

Indication: Any capsular hypomobility.

Subtalar

Compression

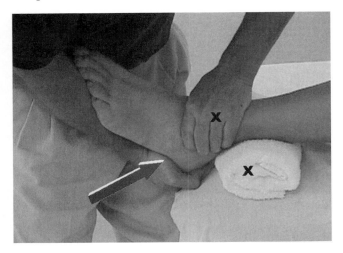

Patient Position: Patient lies supine with the ankle over the edge of the table midway between supination and pronation (LPP).

Therapist Position: Therapist stands facing the patient's foot.

Stabilization: Therapist's cephalic hand grasps the distal leg and talus on the medial and lateral sides.

Mobilization: Therapist's caudal hand cups the calcaneus in the palm of the hand.

Direction of Force: Therapist compresses the calcaneus in a cephalic and anterior direction.

Indication: Provocation findings with arthritis.[1]

Subtalar

Medial Glide

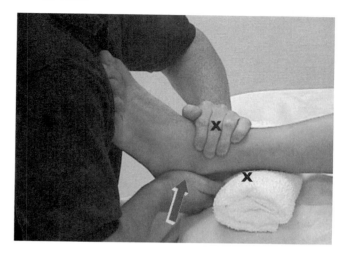

Patient Position: Patient lies supine with the knee slightly flexed and the ankle over the edge of the table midway between supination and pronation (LPP).

Therapist Position: Therapist stands facing the patient's foot.

Stabilization: Therapist's thigh or chest presses against the distal aspect of the patient's foot in order to maintain full dorsiflexion fixating the talus between the tibia and fibula. Therapist's medial hand grasps the distal leg and talus posteriorly and medially.

Mobilization: Therapist's lateral hand grasps the calcaneus on the lateral side.

Direction of Force: Therapist glides the calcaneus in a medial direction.

Indication: Eversion hypomobility.

Subtalar

Lateral Glide

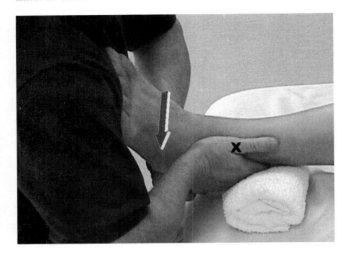

Patient Position: Patient lies supine with the knee slightly flexed and the ankle over the edge of the table midway between supination and pronation (LPP).

Therapist Position: Therapist stands facing the patient's foot.

Stabilization: Therapist's thigh or chest presses against the distal aspect of the patient's foot in order to maintain full dorsiflexion fixating the talus between the tibia and fibula. Therapist's lateral hand grasps the distal leg and talus posteriorly and laterally.

Mobilization: Therapist's medial hand grasps the calcaneus on the medial side.

Direction of Force: Therapist glides the calcaneus in a lateral direction.

Indication: Inversion hypomobility.

Navicular/Talus

Dorsal Glide

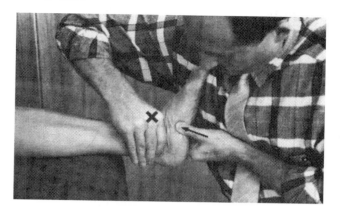

Patient Position: Patient lies supine with the knee extended and the ankle/foot over the edge of the table in a midrange position.

Therapist Position: Therapist sits or stands facing the plantar aspect of the patient's foot.

Stabilization: Therapist's chest stabilizes the caudal aspect of the patient's foot. Therapist's cephalic hand grasps the dorsal surface of the talus between the thumb and index finger.

Mobilization: Therapist's caudal hand (thumb or hypothenar eminence) is placed on the plantar surface of the navicular.

Direction of Force: Therapist glides the navicular in a dorsal direction.

Indication: Pronation hypomobility.

Cuneiforms/Navicular

Dorsal Glide

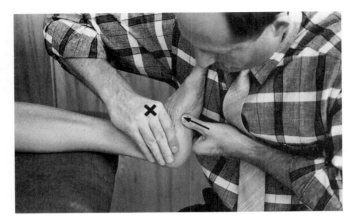

Patient Position: Patient lies supine with the knee extended and the ankle/foot over the edge of the table in a midrange position.

Therapist Position: Therapist sits or stands facing the plantar aspect of the patient's foot.

Stabilization: Therapist's chest stabilizes the caudal aspect of the patient's foot. Therapist's cephalic hand grasps the dorsal surface of the navicular between the thumb and index finger.

Mobilization: Therapist's caudal hand (thumb or hypothenar eminence) is placed on the plantar surface of the three cuneiforms.

Direction of Force: Therapist glides the cuneiforms in a dorsal direction.

Indication: Pronation hypomobility.

Cuboid/Navicular-Cuneiform III

Dorsal Glide

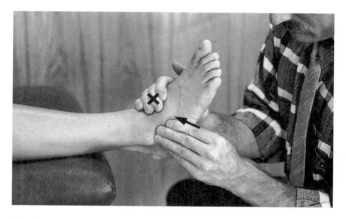

Patient Position: Patient lies supine with the knee extended and the ankle/foot over the edge of the table in a midrange position.

Therapist Position: Therapist sits or stands facing the plantar aspect of the patient's foot.

Stabilization: Therapist's medial hand grasps the dorsal surfaces of the navicular and cuneiform III.

Mobilization: Therapist's lateral hand (thumb or hypothenar eminence) is placed over the plantar aspect of the cuboid.

Direction of Force: Therapist glides the cuboid in a dorsal direction.

Indication: Pronation hypomobility.

Metatarsal I-III/Cuneiform I-III

Dorsal Glide

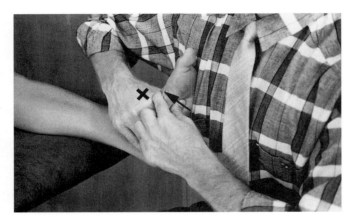

Patient Position: Patient lies supine with the knee extended and the ankle/foot over the edge of the table in a midrange position.

Therapist Position: Therapist sits or stands facing the plantar aspect of the patient's foot.

Stabilization: Therapist's lateral hand grasps the dorsal surface of cuneiform I.

Mobilization: Therapist's medial hand (thumb or hypothenar eminence) is placed on the plantar aspect of the base of metatarsal I.

Direction of Force: Therapist glides metatarsal I in a dorsal direction.

Indication: Pronation hypomobility.

The same technique is applied to metatarsal II stabilizing cuneiforms I–III and metatarsal III stabilizing cuneiform III.

Metatarsal IV-V/Cuboid

Dorsal Glide

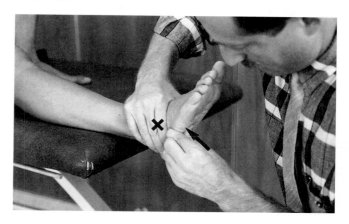

Patient Position: Patient lies supine with the knee extended and the ankle/foot over the edge of the table in a midrange position.

Therapist Position: Therapist sits or stands facing the plantar aspect of the patient's foot.

Stabilization: Therapist's cephalic hand grasps the dorsal surface of the cuboid.

Mobilization: Therapist's caudal hand (thumb or hypothenar eminence) is placed over the plantar aspect of the base of metatarsals IV and V (both can be assessed together or individually).

Direction of Force: Therapist glides metatarsals IV and V in a dorsal direction.

Indication: Pronation hypomobility.

Cuboid/Calcaneus

Dorsal Glide

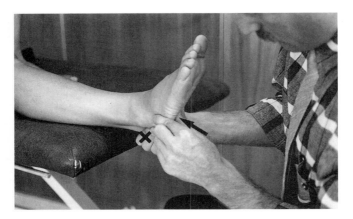

Patient Position: Patient lies supine with the knee extended and the ankle/foot over the edge of the table in a midrange position.

Therapist Position: Therapist sits or stands facing the plantar aspect of the patient's foot.

Stabilization: Therapist's medial hand grasps the calcaneus.

Mobilization: Therapist's lateral hand (thumb or hypothenar eminence) grasps the plantar aspect of the cuboid.

Direction of Force: Therapist glides the cuboid in a dorsal direction.

Indication: Supination hypomobility.

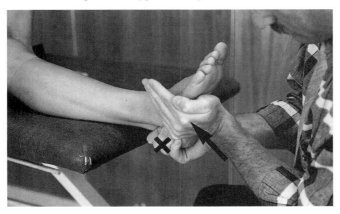

Navicular/Talus

Plantar Glide

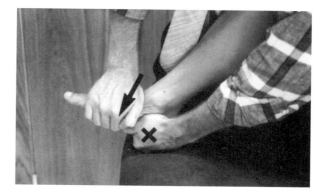

Patient Position: Patient lies supine with the knee flexed, the forefoot over the edge of the table, and the ankle/foot in a midrange position.

Therapist Position: Therapist stands lateral to the foot supporting the patient's leg with his/her proximal arm and trunk.

Stabilization: Therapist's cephalic hand grasps the calcaneus around the plantar surface or uses a wedge under the calcaneus.

Mobilization: Therapist's caudal hand (thumb or thenar eminence) is placed over the dorsal aspect of the navicular.

Direction of Force: Therapist glides the navicular in a plantar direction.

Indication: Supination hypomobility.

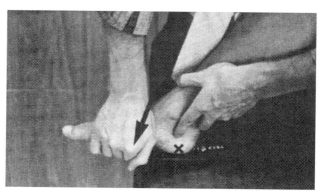

Plantar Glide with Wedge

Cuneiforms/Navicular

Plantar Glide

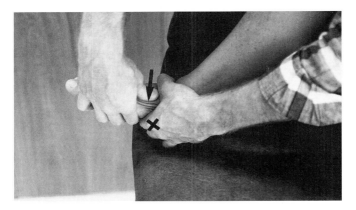

Patient Position: Patient lies supine with the knee flexed, the forefoot over the edge of the table, and the ankle/foot in a midrange position.

Therapist Position: Therapist stands lateral to the foot supporting the patient's leg with his/her proximal arm and trunk.

Stabilization: Therapist's cephalic hand grasps the plantar surface of the navicular.

Mobilization: Therapist's caudal hand, thumb (figure above) or thenar eminence (figure below), is placed over the dorsal aspect of the three cuneiforms.

Direction of Force: Therapist glides the cuneiforms in a plantar direction.

Indication: Supination hypomobility.

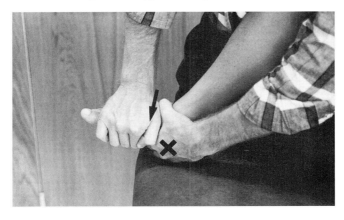

Cuboid/Navicular-Cuneiform III

Plantar Glide

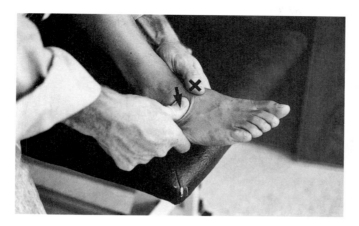

Patient Position: Patient lies supine with the knee flexed, the forefoot over the edge of the table, and the ankle/foot in a midrange position.

Therapist Position: Therapist stands lateral to the foot supporting the patient's leg with his/her proximal arm and trunk.

Stabilization: Therapist's medial hand grasps the plantar surface of the navicular and cuneiform III.

Mobilization: Therapist's lateral hand, thumb (figure above) or thenar eminence (not pictured), is placed on the dorsal aspect of the cuboid.

Direction of Force: Therapist glides the cuboid in a plantar direction.

Indication: Supination hypomobility.

Metatarsals I–III/Cuneiforms I–III

Plantar Glide

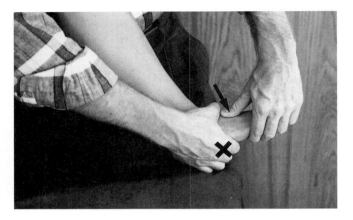

Patient Position: Patient lies supine with the knee flexed, the forefoot over the edge of the table, and the ankle/foot in a midrange position.

Therapist Position: Therapist stands lateral to the foot supporting the patient's leg with the therapist's proximal arm and trunk.

Stabilization: Therapist's cephalic hand grasps cuneiform I on the plantar surface.

Mobilization: Therapist's caudal hand, thumb (figure above) or thenar eminence (not pictured), is placed on the dorsal aspect of metatarsal I.

Direction of Force: Therapist glides metatarsal I in a plantar direction.

Indication: Supination hypomobility.

The same technique is applied to metatarsal II stabilizing cuneiforms I–III and metatarsal III stabilizing cuneiform III.

Metatarsal IV-V/Cuboid

Plantar Glide

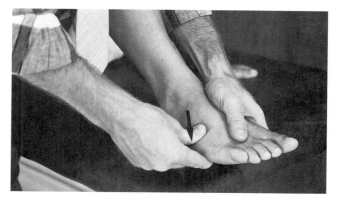

Patient Position: Patient lies supine with the knee flexed, the forefoot over the edge of the table, and the ankle/foot in a midrange position.

Therapist Position: Therapist stands lateral to the foot supporting the patient's leg with his/her proximal arm and trunk.

Stabilization: Therapist's medial hand grasps the plantar surface of the cuboid.

Mobilization: Therapist's lateral hand (thumb or hypothenar eminence) is placed over the dorsal aspect of the base of metatarsal IV and V (both can be assessed together or individually.

Direction of Force: Therapist glides metatarsal IV and V in a plantar direction.

Indication: Supination hypomobility.

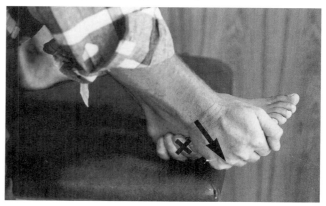

Cuboid/Calcaneus

Plantar Glide

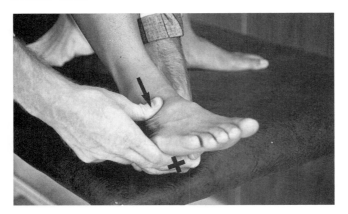

Patient Position: Patient lies supine with the knee flexed, the forefoot over the edge of the table, and the ankle/foot in a midrange position.

Therapist Position: Therapist stands lateral to the foot supporting the patient's leg with his/her proximal arm and trunk.

Stabilization: Therapist's medial hand grasps the plantar surface of the calcaneus.

Mobilization: Therapist's lateral hand (thumb or hypothenar eminence) is placed over the dorsal aspect of the cuboid.

Direction of Force: Therapist glides the cuboid in a plantar direction.

Indication: Pronation hypomobility.

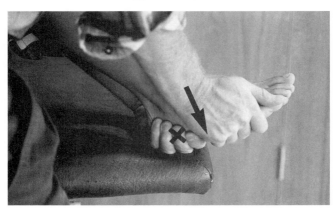

Intermetatarsal I–V

Dorsal/Plantar Glides

Patient Position: Patient lies supine with the knee flexed and the forefoot over the edge of the table.

Therapist Position: Therapist stands facing the patient's toes.

Stabilization: Therapist stabilizes the metatarsals using a lumbrical grip.

Mobilization: Therapist grasps a specific metatarsal between the thumb and forefinger (top figure, next page) or uses a lumbrical grip (bottom figure, next page).

Direction of Force: Therapist glides the specific metatarsal in a plantar or dorsal direction on the stabilized metatarsals.

Indications: Pronation hypomobility (dorsal) and supination hypomobility (plantar).

The second metatarsal is considered the stable ray.

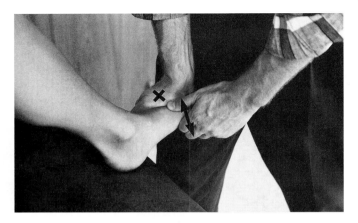

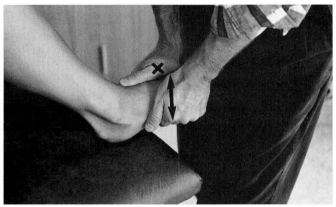

Metatarsophalangeal I–V/Interphalangeal I–V

Distraction

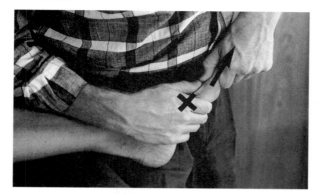

Patient Position: Patient lies supine with the metatarsophalangeal joint in slight extension or the interphalangeal joint in slight flexion (LPP).

Therapist Position: Therapist stands along the lateral side of the patient's foot.

Stabilization: Therapist's cephalic hand grasps the dorsal and volar surfaces of the metatarsal.

Mobilization: Therapist's caudal hand grasps the dorsal and volar surfaces of the proximal phalanx.

Direction of Force: Therapist distracts the proximal phalanx from the metatarsal.

Indication: Any capsular hypomobility.

The same technique is applied to all the interphalangeal joints.

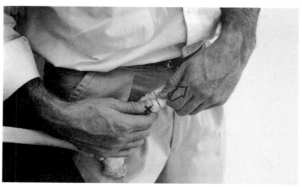

Skeletal Metatarsophalangeal Distraction

Metatarsophalangeal I–V/Interphalangeal I–V

Compression

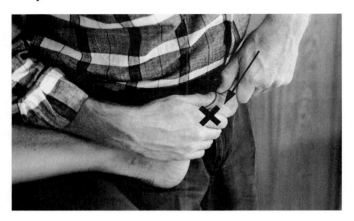

Patient Position: Patient lies supine with the metatarsophalangeal joint in slight extension or the interphalangeal joint in slight flexion (LPP).

Therapist Position: Therapist stands along the lateral side of the patient's foot.

Stabilization: Therapist's cephalic hand grasps the dorsal and volar surfaces of the metatarsal.

Mobilization: Therapist's caudal hand grasps the dorsal and volar surfaces of the proximal phalanx.

Direction of Force: Therapist compresses the proximal phalanx into the metatarsal.

Indication: Provocation finding with arthritis.[1]

The same technique is applied to all the interphalangeal joints.

Metatarsophalangeal I–V/Interphalangeal I–V

Dorsal Glide

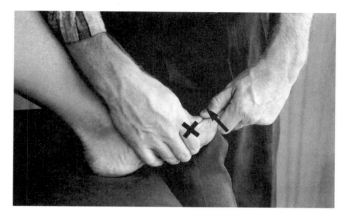

Patient Position: Patient lies supine with the metatarsophalangeal joint in slight extension or the interphalangeal joint in slight flexion (LPP).

Therapist Position: Therapist stands along the lateral side of the patient's foot.

Stabilization: Therapist's cephalic hand grasps the dorsal and volar surfaces of the metatarsal.

Mobilization: Therapist's caudal hand grasps the dorsal and volar surfaces of the proximal phalanx.

Direction of Force: Therapist glides the proximal phalanx in a dorsal direction.

Indication: Extension hypomobility.

The same technique is applied to all the interphalangeal joints.

Metatarsophalangeal I–V/Interphalangeal I–V

Plantar Glide

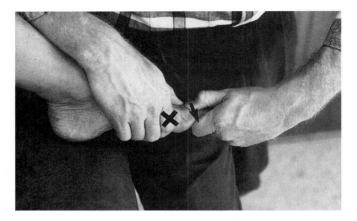

Patient Position: Patient lies supine with the metatarsophalangeal joint in slight extension or the interphalangeal joint in slight flexion (LPP).

Therapist Position: Therapist stands along the lateral side of the patient's foot.

Stabilization: Therapist's cephalic hand grasps the dorsal and volar surfaces of the metatarsal.

Mobilization: Therapist's caudal hand grasps the dorsal and volar surfaces of the proximal phalanx.

Direction of Force: Therapist glides the proximal phalanx in a plantar direction.

Indication: Flexion hypomobility.

The same technique is applied to all the interphalangeal joints.

Metatarsophalangeal I–V/Interphalangeal I–V

Medial Glide

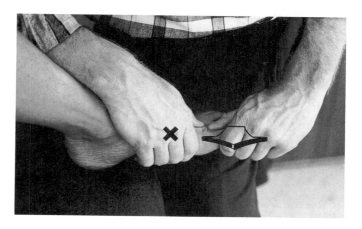

Patient Position: Patient lies supine with the metatarsophalangeal joint in slight extension or the interphalangeal joint in slight flexion (LPP).

Therapist Position: Therapist stands along the lateral side of the patient's foot.

Stabilization: Therapist's cephalic hand grasps the medial and lateral surfaces of the metatarsal.

Mobilization: Therapist's caudal hand grasps the medial and lateral surfaces of the proximal phalanx.

Direction of Force: Therapist glides the proximal phalanx in a medial direction.

Indications: I & II abduction hypomobility and III to V adduction hypomobility.

The same technique is applied to all the interphalangeal joints.

Metatarsophalangeal I–V/Interphalangeal I–V

Lateral Glide

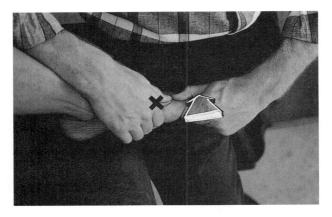

Patient Position: Patient lies supine with the metatarsophalangeal joint in slight extension or the interphalangeal joint in slight flexion (LPP).

Therapist Position: Therapist stands along the lateral side of the patient's foot.

Stabilization: Therapist's cephalic hand grasps the medial and lateral surfaces of the metatarsal.

Mobilization: Therapist's caudal hand grasps the medial and lateral surfaces of the proximal phalanx.

Direction of Force: Therapist glides the proximal phalanx in a lateral direction.

Indications: I & II adduction hypomobility and III to V abduction hypomobility.

The same technique is applied to all the interphalangeal joints.

Metatarsophalangeal I–V/Interphalangeal I–V

Medial Rotation

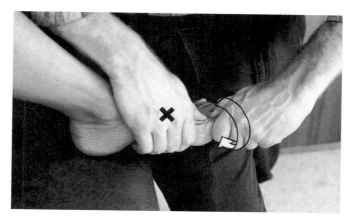

Patient Position: Patient lies supine with the metatarsophalangeal joint in slight extension or the interphalangeal joint in slight flexion (LPP).

Therapist Position: Therapist stands along the lateral side of the patient's foot.

Stabilization: Therapist's cephalic hand grasps the dorsal and volar surfaces of the metatarsal.

Mobilization: Therapist's caudal hand grasps the dorsal and volar surfaces of the proximal phalanx.

Direction of Force: Therapist rotates the proximal phalanx in a medial direction.

Indication: Extension hypomobility.

The same technique is applied to all the interphalangeal joints.

Metatarsophalangeal I–V/Interphalangeal I–V

Lateral Rotation

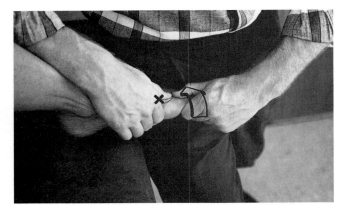

Patient Position: Patient lies supine with the metatarsophalangeal joint in slight extension or the interphalangeal joint in slight flexion (LPP).

Therapist Position: Therapist stands along the lateral side of the patient's foot.

Stabilization: Therapist's cephalic hand grasps the dorsal and volar surfaces of the metatarsal.

Mobilization: Therapist's caudal hand grasps the dorsal and volar surfaces of the proximal phalanx.

Direction of Force: Therapist rotates the proximal phalanx in a lateral direction.

Indication: Flexion hypomobility.

The same technique is applied to all the interphalangeal joints.

NEURODYNAMIC BASE TESTS

Principles of Neurodynamic Base Testing

Performance of base test movements will lead to a variety of responses by the patient. The quantity, quality of movement, end-feel, and the sequence of pain and resistance should be assessed following each movement component. The series of movements that comprise each base test are performed only to the initial point in the range of motion where symptoms are reproduced.

Neurodynamic Base Test

Neck Flexion

Patient Position: Patient lies supine in a neutral position.

Therapist Position: Therapist stands alongside the patient's head.

Stabilization: Provided by the patient's body weight and the therapist's caudal hand on the patient's sternum.

Mobilization: Therapist's cephalic hand cradles the patient's occiput.

Direction of Force: Therapist passively flexes the patient's cervical spine. Additional forces can be added at the hip and/or ankle.

Indications: Provocation findings of thoracic or lumbar symptoms may be suggestive of pons, cord, or meninges involvement.

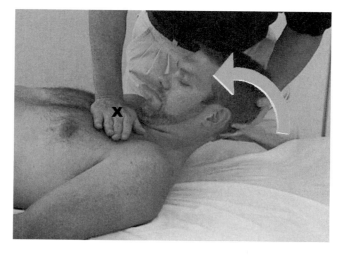

Neurodynamic Base Test

Straight Leg Raise

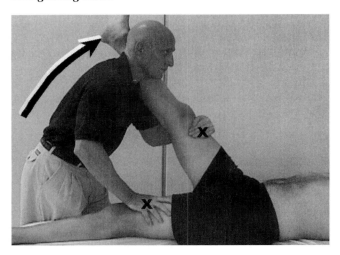

Patient Position: Patient lies supine in a neutral position.

Therapist Position: Therapist stands facing the patient's head along the side to be tested.

Stabilization: Provided by the patient's body weight and the therapist's cephalic hand, which maintains knee extension as the patient's leg rests on the therapist's shoulder.

Mobilization: The therapist's cephalic hand grasps the patient's thigh just above the knee to maintain knee extension.

Direction of Force: Therapist flexes the hip maintaining knee extension. Additional forces can be added at the hip and/or ankle.

Indications: Provocation of lumbar or lower extremity symptoms may be suggestive of meninges, cord, lumbar sympathetic trunk, lumbar nerve root, or lower extremity peripheral nerve involvement.

Neurodynamic Base Test

Slump Test

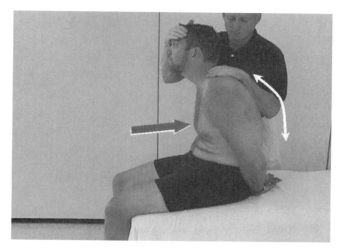

Initial Slump Test Positioning

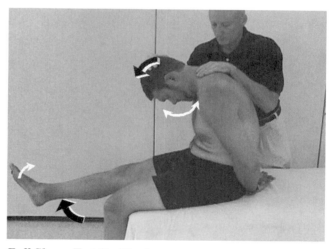

Full Slump Test Positioning

Patient Position: Patient sits with his/her hands behind his/her back maintaining a vertical pelvis.

Therapist Position: Therapist stands alongside the patient.

Stabilization: Provided by the patient's body weight and the therapist's caudal hand.

Mobilization: Sequentially the following movements are added: (a) the patient slumps with his/her cervical spine neutral; (b) the patient flexes his/her cervical spine and the therapist maintains this position with light pressure (top figure page 225); (c) the patient extends one knee; (d) the patient dorsiflexes his/her ankle (bottom figure page 225); (e) the patient releases cervical flexion (a sensitizing maneuver). The same procedure is repeated for the opposite leg.

Indications: Provocation of lumbar or lower extremity symptoms may be suggestive of pons, meninges, cord, or sciatic nerve involvement.

Neurodynamic Base Test

Femoral Nerve

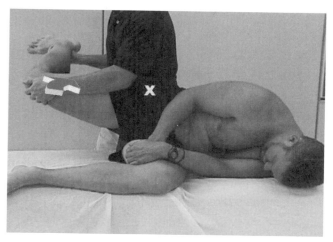

Patient Position: Patient is side-lying in cervical and lumbar flexion, maintaining one hip in flexion.

Therapist Position: Therapist stands facing the patient's back.

Stabilization: Provided by the patient's body weight and by the therapist's body next to the patient's pelvis.

Mobilization: Therapist passively extends the patient's hip while maintaining the knee flexed.

Indications: Provocation of lumbar or lower extremity symptoms may be suggestive of meninges, cord, lumbar nerve root, or femoral nerve involvement.

Neurodynamic Base Test

Median Nerve (Elvey Test)

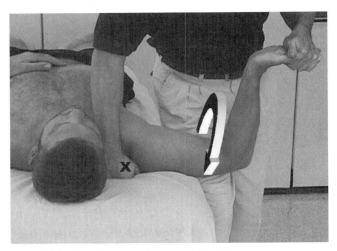

Initial Median Nerve (Elvey Test) Positioning

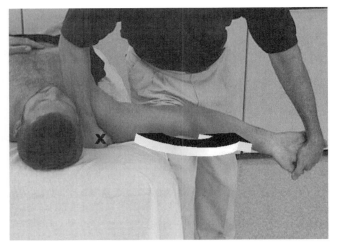

Full Median Nerve (Elvey Test) Positioning

Patient Position: Patient lies supine in a neutral position.

Therapist Position: Therapist stands facing the patient on the side to be examined.

Stabilization: Provided by the patient's body weight and the therapist's cephalic hand prevents scapular elevation.

Mobilization: Sequentially the following movements are added: (a) shoulder abduction; (b) forearm supination; (c) wrist/finger/thumb extension (top figure page 228); (d) shoulder external rotation; (e) elbow extension (bottom figure page 228); and (f) cervical lateral flexion (ipsilateral and contralateral as a sensitizing maneuver).

Indications: Provocation of cervical, thoracic, or upper extremity symptoms may be suggestive of cervical or thoracic nerve root or median nerve involvement.

Neurodynamic Base Test

Median Nerve

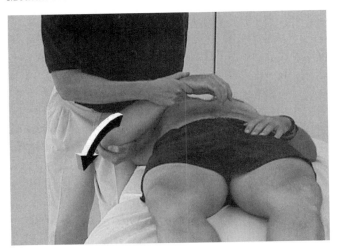

Initial Median Nerve Positioning

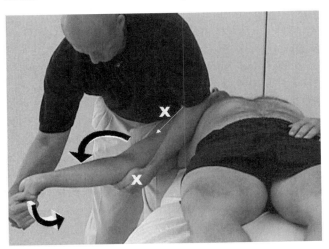

Full Median Nerve Positioning

Patient Position: Patient lies supine in a neutral position with the shoulder to be tested at the edge of the table.

Therapist Position: Therapist stands at the head of the patient on the side to be examined.

Stabilization: Provided by the patient's body weight and by the therapist's hip that maintains full scapular depression.

Mobilization: Sequentially the following movements are added: (a) elbow extension; (b) shoulder internal rotation; (c) forearm supination; (d) wrist/finger/thumb extension; (e) shoulder abduction; and (f) cervical lateral flexion (ipsilateral and contralateral as a sensitizing maneuver).

Indications: Provocation of cervical or upper extremity symptoms may be suggestive of cervical or thoracic nerve root or median nerve involvement.

Neurodynamic Base Test

Radial Nerve

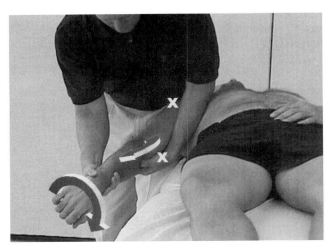

Initial Radial Nerve Positioning

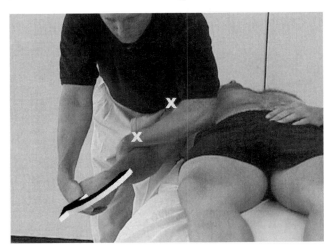

Full Ulnar Nerve Positioning

Patient Position: Patient lies supine in a neutral position with the shoulder to be tested at the edge of the table.

Therapist Position: Therapist stands at the head of the patient on the side to be examined.

Stabilization: Stabilization is provided by the patient's body weight and by the therapist's hip which maintains full scapular depression.

Mobilization: Sequentially the following movements are added: (a) elbow extension; (b) shoulder internal rotation; (c) forearm pronation (top figure page 232); (d) wrist/finger/thumb flexion with ulnar deviation; (e) shoulder abduction (bottom figure page 232); and (f) cervical lateral flexion (ipsilateral and contralateral as a sensitizing maneuver).

Indications: Provocation of cervical or upper extremity symptoms may be suggestive of cervical or thoracic nerve root or radial nerve involvement.

Neurodynamic Base Test

Ulnar Nerve

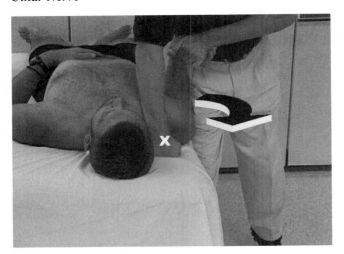

Initial Ulnar Nerve Positioning

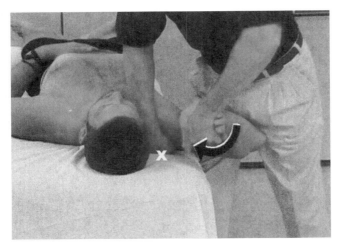

Full Ulnar Nerve Positioning

Patient Position: Patient lies supine in a neutral position.

Therapist Position: Therapist stands facing the patient on the side to be examined.

Stabilization: Provided by the patient's body weight and the therapist's cephalic hand prevents scapular elevation.

Mobilization: Sequentially the following movements are added: (a) finger/wrist extension; (b) forearm pronation; (c) elbow flexion; (d) scapula depression (top figure page 234); (e) shoulder external rotation; (f) shoulder abduction (bottom figure page 234); and (g) cervical lateral flexion (ipsilateral and contralateral as a sensitizing maneuver).

Indications: Provocation of cervical or upper extremity symptoms may be suggestive of cervical or thoracic nerve root or ulnar nerve involvement.

PELVIS, SPINE, AND TEMPOROMANDIBULAR JOINT

Sacroiliac

Physiologic Movement Testing: Standing Flexion Test

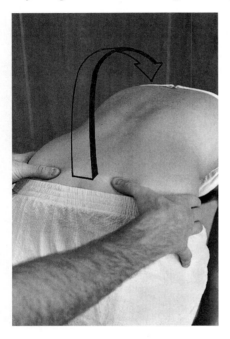

Patient Position: Patient stands with the lower extremities approximately shoulder width apart and feet parallel to each other.

Therapist Position: Therapist stands behind the patient so that the therapist's eyes are at the level of the patient's posterior superior iliac spines.

Stabilization: Provided by the patient's body weight.

Mobilization: Therapist places thumbs firmly over the posterior superior iliac spines of the patient.

Direction of Force: Patient forward bends as far as possible keeping the knees straight. Therapist monitors the posterior superior iliac spine's positions through the full range of motion.

Indication: Motion of one posterior superior iliac spine more superiorly or prematurely compared with the opposite side suggests the possibility of iliosacral hypomobility. The side that moves more superiorly is purported to be the hypomobile side.[5;6]

Sacroiliac

Physiologic Movement Testing: Standing Backward Bending

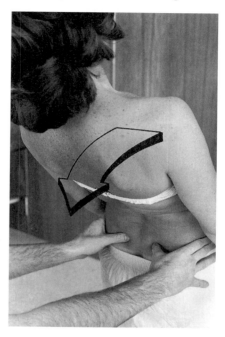

Patient Position: Patient stands in a neutral spinal posture.

Therapist Position: Therapist stands behind the patient so that therapist's eyes are at the level of the patient's sacral sulci.

Stabilization: Provided by the patient's body weight and if necessary the patient may lean against a table.

Mobilization: Therapist places thumbs firmly over the sacral sulci of the patient.

Direction of Force: Patient backward bends as far as possible. Therapist monitors the sacral sulci position through the full range of motion. Comparison is made from one side to the other.

Indication: The sacral sulci should become more shallow during backward bending.

Sacroiliac

Physiologic Movement Testing: March Test

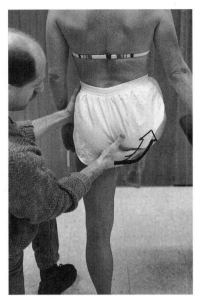

Ischial Tuberosity Palpation

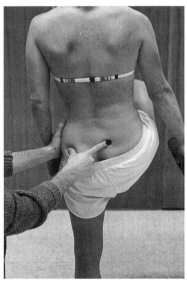

*Posterior Superior Iliac
Spine Palpation*

Patient Position: Patient stands with legs approximately shoulder width apart and feet parallel.

Therapist Position: Therapist kneels behind the patient.

Stabilization: Therapist's hand stabilizes the contralateral hip/pelvis while the patient grasps the edge of the treatment table for balance.

Mobilization: Therapist palpates the posterior superior iliac spine or ischial tuberosity with the other hand.

Direction of Force: Patient maximally flexes the ipsilateral hip and the therapist monitors the position of the posterior superior iliac spine or ischial tuberosity. Comparison of motion is made to the opposite side.

Indication: Asymmetry of motion from right to left sides is suggestive of possible iliosacral dysfunction. Normal movement of the posterior superior iliac spine or the ischial tuberosity is in an inferior and lateral direction.

Sacroiliac

Physiologic Movement Testing: Sitting Flexion Test

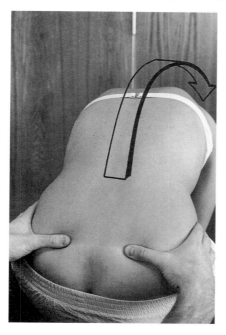

Patient Position: Patient sits near the edge of the table with his/her feet supported on a stool (or floor) and legs abducted comfortably.

Therapist Position: Therapist stands behind the patient with the therapist's eyes at the level of the patient's posterior superior iliac spines.

Stabilization: Provided by the patient's body weight.

Mobilization: Therapist places thumbs firmly over the posterior superior iliac spines of the patient.

Direction of Force: Patient bends forward as far as possible. Therapist monitors the position of the posterior superior iliac spines through the full range of motion.

Indication: Motion of one posterior superior iliac spine more superiorly or prematurely compared with the opposite side suggests the possibility of sacroiliac or iliosacral hypomobility.

Sacroiliac

Physiologic Movement Testing: Sitting Backward Bending

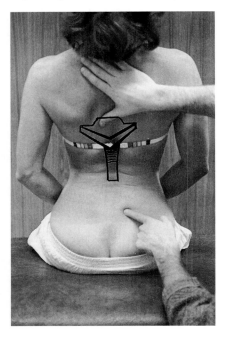

Patient Position: Patient sits in a neutral spinal posture with feet supported.

Therapist Position: Therapist stands behind the patient so the therapist's eyes are at the level of the patient's sacral sulci.

Stabilization: Provided by the patient's body weight, the table, and the therapist.

Mobilization: Therapist places a thumb firmly over the sacral sulcus area on one side of the patient.

Direction of Force: Patient backward bends as far as possible. Therapist monitors the sacral sulcus position through the full range of motion. Comparison is made from one side to the other.

Indication: The sacral sulci should become more shallow during backward bending.

Sacroiliac

Supine/Long Sit Test

Patient Position: Patient begins by lying in the supine position with feet together.

Therapist Position: Therapist stands at the foot of the table positioned over the patient's malleoli.

Stabilization: Provided by the patient's body weight.

Mobilization: Therapist places both thumbs on the inferior aspect of the medial malleoli bilaterally. An initial assessment of symmetry between the malleoli is made in the supine position. Therapist then lifts patient's legs slightly off the table.

Direction of Force: The patient actively moves into a long sitting position. The therapist again palpates the medial malleoli for any change in symmetry in the new position.

Indication: A change of greater than ¼- to ½-inch in length is suggestive of the possibility of iliosacral dysfunction. An initial long leg that shortens suggests an anterior rotation or an initial short leg that lengthens suggests a posterior rotation of the ilium. This test should be repeated several times.

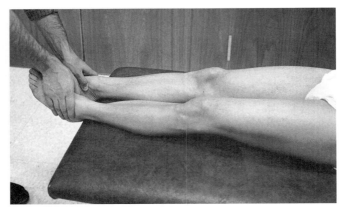

Supine/Long Sit Test Initial Position

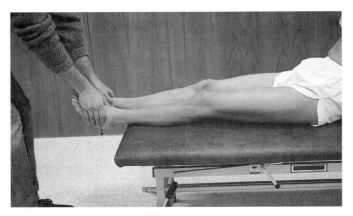

Supine/Long Sit Test Full Position

Sacroiliac

Passive Accessory Movement Testing: Anterior Gap Test

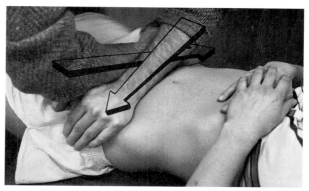

Patient Position: Patient lies supine with legs extended and positioned close to the edge of the table.

Therapist Position: Therapist stands facing the patient leaning directly over the patient's body.

Stabilization: Provided by the patient's body weight and a towel placed under the lumbar spine.

Mobilization: Therapist places the heel of each hand on the medial aspect of the contralateral iliac crest using a crossed forearm position.

Direction of Force: A laterally directed force is produced simultaneously with both hands as if to distract the crests of the ilia away from each other.

Indication: A positive test results if pain is provoked posteriorly suggesting possible sacroiliac or lumbosacral pathology.

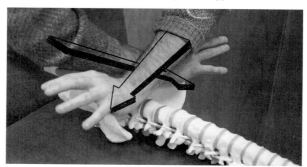

Skeletal Anterior Gap Test

Sacroiliac

Passive Accessory Movement Testing: Posterior Gap Test

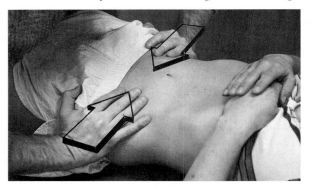

Patient Position: Patient lies supine with legs extended and positioned close to the side of the table.

Therapist Position: Therapist stands facing the patient leaning directly over the patient's body.

Stabilization: Provided by the patient's body weight and a towel placed under the lumbar spine.

Mobilization: Therapist places the heel of each hand over the ipsilateral lateral iliac crest with fingers directed toward the midline.

Direction of Force: An inwardly directed force is produced simultaneously with both hands as if to compress the crests of the ilia together.

Indication: A positive test results if pain is provoked posteriorly suggesting possible sacroiliac or lumbosacral dysfunction.

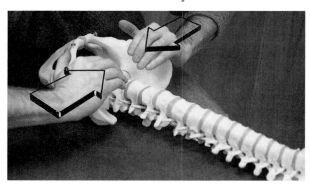

Skeletal Posterior Gap Test

Sacroiliac

Passive Accessory Movement Testing: Hip Flexion/Adduction Gap Test

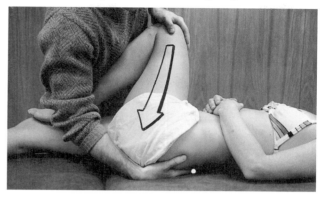

Patient Position: Patient lies supine near the edge of the table.

Therapist Position: Therapist stands near the pelvis facing superiorly.

Stabilization: Provided by the table and the palpation hand under the sacrum.

Mobilization: Therapist flexes the ipsilateral or contralateral hip to 90° and adducts the thigh until a gapping motion is perceived at the sacral sulcus with the palpating hand.

Direction of Force: The therapist produces a longitudinal compression force through the long axis of the femur while palpating at the sacral sulcus. This should produce a posterior glide of the ilium on the sacrum.

Indication: Asymmetry of motion when compared right to left or provocation of symptoms suggests possible sacroiliac or iliosacral pathology.

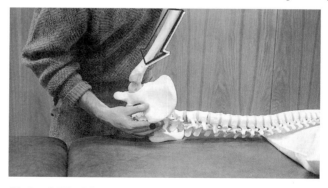

Skeletal Hip Flexion/Adduction Gap Test

Sacroiliac

Passive Accessory Movement Testing: Lower Extremity Rotation Gap

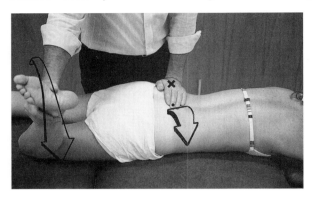

Patient Position: Patient lies prone near the edge of the table.

Therapist Position: Therapist stands facing the patient's pelvis.

Stabilization: Provided by the table and the palpation hand.

Mobilization: Therapist palpates the contralateral sacral sulcus with the proximal hand. The distal hand flexes the contralateral knee to 90°.

Direction of Force: The contralateral femur is internally rotated until motion is perceived with the palpating hand. This movement produces distraction of the contralateral sacral sulcus (ilium on sacrum).

Indication: Asymmetry of motion when compared right to left suggests possible sacroiliac pathology.

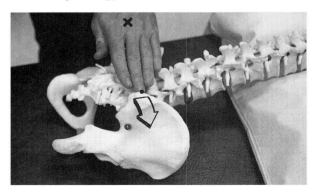

***Skeletal Contralateral Lower Extremity Rotation
Gap Palpation***

Sacroiliac

Passive Accessory Movement Testing: Lower Extremity Rotation Gap

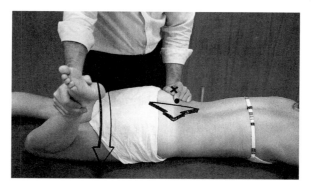

Patient Position: Patient lies prone near the edge of the table.

Therapist Position: Therapist stands facing the patient's pelvis.

Stabilization: Provided by the table and the palpation hand.

Mobilization: Therapist palpates the ipsilateral sacral sulcus with the proximal hand. The distal hand flexes the contralateral knee to 90°.

Direction of Force: The contralateral femur is internally rotated until motion is perceived with the palpating hand. This movement produces distraction of the ipsilateral sacral sulcus (sacrum on ilium).

Indication: Asymmetry of motion when compared right to left suggests possible sacroiliac pathology.

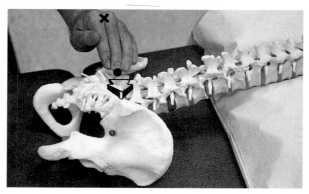

Skeletal Ipsilateral Lower Extremity Rotation Gap Palpation

Sacroiliac

Passive Accessory Movement Testing: Ilial Posterior-Anterior Pressure

Patient Position: Patient lies prone near the edge of the table.

Therapist Position: Therapist stands directly over the patient facing the pelvis.

Stabilization: Therapist's proximal hand is placed directly on the sacrum with the fingers pointing distally.

Mobilization: The heel of the therapist's distal hand is placed on the contralateral posterior superior iliac spine with the fingers around the ilium laterally.

Direction of Force: Therapist glides the ilium in an anterior and lateral direction on the sacrum (see figures on page 249).

Indication: Posterior ilial rotation hypomobility.

Direction of Force: Ilial anterior-posterior pressure can be performed by the same procedure except that the therapist glides the ilium in a posterior and medial direction on the sacrum (not pictured).

Indication: Anterior ilial rotation hypomobility.

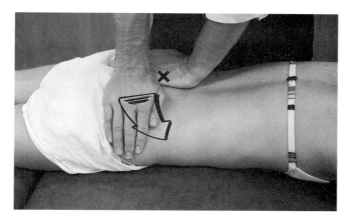

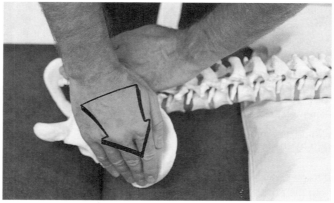

Skeletal Ilial Posterior-Anterior Pressure

Sacroiliac

Passive Accessory Movement Testing: Unilateral Sacral Posterior-Anterior Pressure

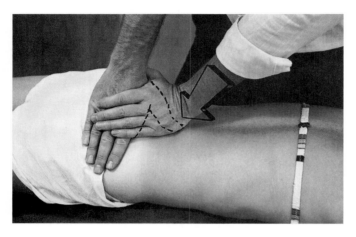

Patient Position: Patient lies prone near the edge of the table.

Therapist Position: Therapist stands directly over the patient facing the pelvis.

Stabilization: Provided by the table.

Mobilization: The therapist's distal thumb is placed on the contralateral side of the sacrum medial to the posterior superior iliac spine (sacral sulcus) (figure above and top figure page 251). The hypothenar eminence of the proximal hand is placed on the thumb (figure above and bottom figure page 251).

Direction of Force: Therapist glides the sacrum in an anterior direction on the ilium (figure above and bottom figure page 251).

Indication: Counternutation hypomobility.

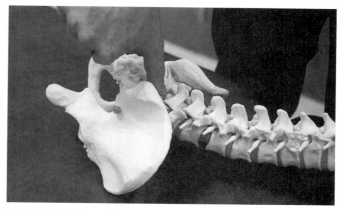

Skeletal Unilateral Sacral Posterior-Anterior
Thumb Positioning

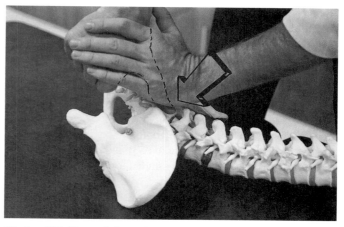

Skeletal Unilateral Sacral Posterior-Anterior Hypothenar
Eminence Positioning

Sacroiliac

Passive Accessory Movement Testing: Unilateral Posterior-Anterior Pressure L5

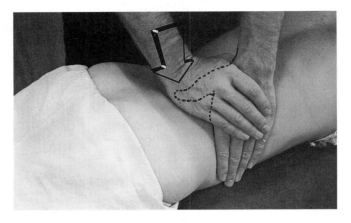

Patient Position: Patient lies prone near the edge of the table.

Therapist Position: Therapist stands directly over the patient facing the lumbosacral junction.

Stabilization: Provided by the patient's body weight and the table.

Mobilization: Therapist places the proximal thumb onto the contralateral L5 transverse process (figure above and top figure page 253) and covers the thumb with the hypothenar eminence of the distal hand (figure above and bottom figure page 253).

Direction of Force: Therapist glides the L5 transverse process in an anterior direction (figure above and bottom figure page 253).

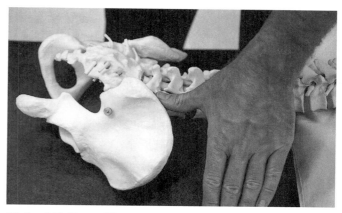

Skeletal Unilateral Posterior-Anterior Pressure L5 Palpation

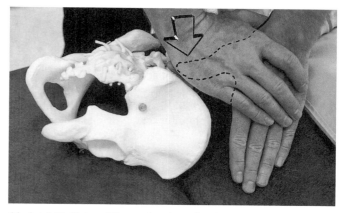

Skeletal Unilateral Posterior-Anterior Pressure L5 with Hypothenar Eminence

Coccyx

Passive Accessory Movement Testing: Posterior-Anterior Pressure

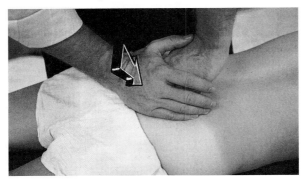

Patient Position: Patient lies prone near the edge of the table.

Therapist Position: Therapist stands directly over the patient facing the sacro-coccygeal region.

Stabilization: Provided by the patient's body weight and the table.

Mobilization: Therapist places the index finger of the proximal hand on the coccyx and covers the finger with the hypothenar eminence of the distal hand.

Direction of Force: Therapist moves the coccyx in an anterior direction on the sacrum.

Indication: Flexion hypomobility.

Direction of Force: Mobilization of the coccyx in a posterior direction on the sacrum can be done internally through the anus (not pictured).

Indication: Extension hypomobility.

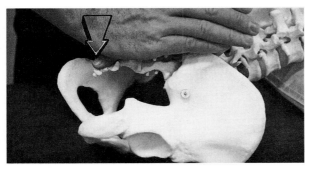

Skeletal Coccyx Posterior-Anterior Pressure

Coccyx

Passive Accessory Movement Testing: Transverse Pressure

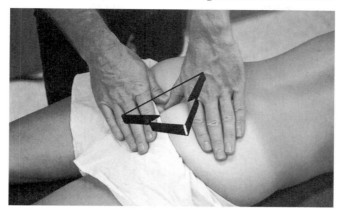

Patient Position: Patient lies prone near the edge of the table.

Therapist Position: Therapist stands directly over the patient facing the sacro-coccygeal region.

Stabilization: Provided by the patient's body weight and the table.

Mobilization: Therapist places the thumb of the proximal hand on the ipsilateral side of the coccyx and covers the thumb with the distal thumb.

Direction of Force: Therapist moves the coccyx in a lateral direction.

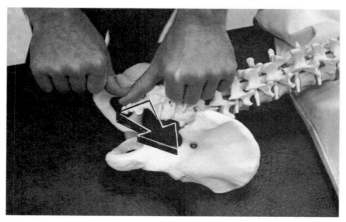

Skeletal Coccyx Transverse Pressure

Trunk

Axial Compression Testing

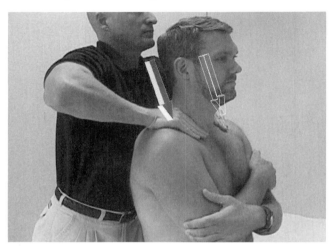

Patient Position: Patient sits in a neutral spine position with the feet supported.

Therapist Position: Therapist stands behind the patient.

Stabilization: Provided by the patient's body weight.

Mobilization: Therapist places each of his/her hands adjacent to the spine on either side of the patient's neck.

Direction of Force: Therapist slowly imparts a downward force on either side of the spine adjacent to the patient's neck, compressing the cervical-thoracic junction, thoracic and lumbar spines for 3 to 5 seconds, and then releasing slowly. It is important not to allow movement of the trunk during this test.

Indications: Reproduction of symptoms makes this a positive test for weight-bearing structures. Occasionally this test will alleviate symptoms as well.

Trunk

Axial Decompression Testing (Traction)

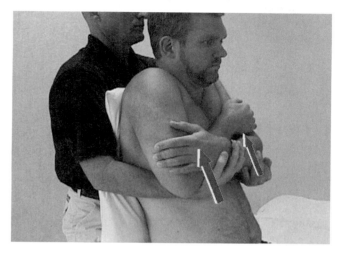

Patient Position: Patient sits in a neutral spine posture with his/her arms crossed over his/her chest with the feet supported.

Therapist Position: Therapist stands behind the patient.

Stabilization: Provided by the patient's body weight and the therapist's body. A pillow placed between the therapist and patient may be used to support the patient.

Mobilization: Therapist grasps under/around each of the patient's elbow/forearm areas.

Direction of Force: Therapist lifts cephalically with both hands.

Indications: A change in symptoms makes this a positive test for weight-bearing or ligamentous structures.

Lumbar (T11/12–L5/S1)

Active Movement Testing/Overpressure: Forward Bending

Observe the patient standing or sitting from an anterior, a posterior, and both lateral views. Note any asymmetries using major landmarks and differences in the two positions.

Patient Position: Patient stands in neutral posture and then bends forward as far as possible (top figure, page 259).

Therapist Position: Stand and observe the patient's active movement. The therapist stands alongside facing the patient for the overpressure.

Stabilization: The therapist's body alongside the patient provides stabilization during the overpressure.

Mobilization: The therapist's forearms are placed one across the upper thoracic region and the other across the ischial tuberosities during the overpressure.

Direction of Force: Therapist's forearms bow the lumbar spine into forward bending for an overpressure (bottom figure, page 259).

Ask questions regarding the reproduction of symptoms while observing the quality and quantity of active movements. Assess the movements from the top down, noting segmental recruitment of motion. Identify deviations from the normal planes of motion including rotation, side bending, forward, or backward bending.

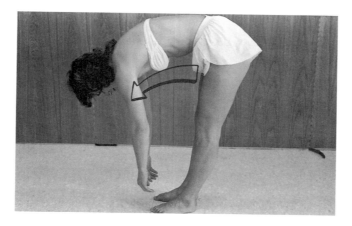

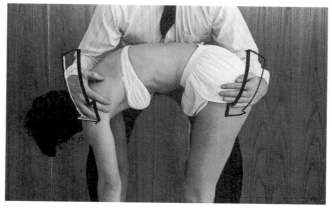

Lumbar Forward Bending Overpressure

Lumbar (T11/12-L5/S1)

Active Movement Testing/Overpressure: Backward Bending

Observe the patient standing or sitting from an anterior, a posterior, and both lateral views. Note any asymmetries using major landmarks and differences in the two positions.

Patient Position: Patient stands in neutral posture with hands on his/her buttocks and then bends back as far as possible (bottom figures page 261).

Therapist Position: Stand and observe the patient's active movement. The therapist stands behind the patient during the overpressure.

Stabilization: When necessary the patient's anterior pelvis may rest against a nonmovable table.

Mobilization: The therapist's hands are positioned over the upper trapezii as close to the spine as possible during the overpressure.

Direction of Force: Therapist bows the lumbar spine into backward bending by directing the force down through the hands toward the L5 level for an overpressure (top figure page 261).

Ask questions regarding the reproduction of symptoms while observing the quality and quantity of active movements. Assess the movements from the top down, noting segmental recruitment of motion. Identify deviations from the normal planes of motion including rotation, side bending, forward, or backward bending.

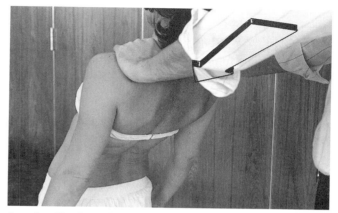

Lumbar Backward Bending Overpressure

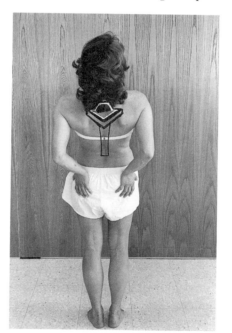

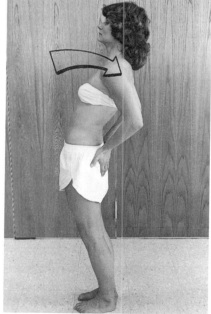

Lumbar Backward Bending Active Movement Testing

Lumbar (T11/12–L5/S1)

Active Movement Testing/Overpressure: Side Bending

Observe the patient standing or sitting from an anterior, a posterior, and both lateral views. Note any asymmetries using major landmarks and differences in the two positions.

Patient Position: Patient stands in neutral posture and then side bends as far as possible (left figure page 263).

Therapist Position: Stand and observe the patient's active movement. The therapist stands alongside and facing the patient during the overpressure.

Stabilization: The therapist's body stabilizes the side of the patient's pelvis during the overpressure.

Mobilization: The therapist places both hands on top of the opposite shoulder during the overpressure.

Direction of Force: Therapist's hands bow the lumbar spine into side bending directing the force to the L5 level for an overpressure (right figure page 263).

Ask questions regarding the reproduction of symptoms while observing the quality and quantity of active movements. Assess the movements from the top down, noting segmental recruitment of motion. Identify deviations from the normal planes of motion including rotation, side bending, forward, or backward bending.

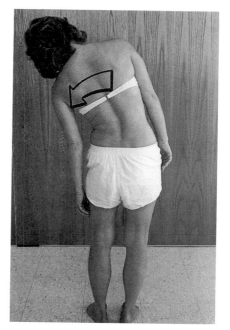 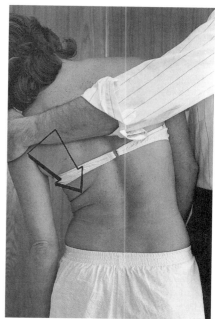

Lumbar Side Bending Active Movement Testing and Overpressure

Lumbar (T11/12–L5/S1)

Active Movement Testing/Overpressure: Rotation

Observe the patient standing or sitting from an anterior, a posterior, and both lateral views. Note any asymmetries using major landmarks and differences in the two positions.

Patient Position: Patient sits in a neutral posture with the upper extremities crossed in the "genie position" and then rotates as far as possible (left figure page 265).

Therapist Position: Stand and observe the patient's active movement from anterior, posterior, and lateral views. The therapist stands facing the patient on the same side the patient rotates toward during the overpressure.

Stabilization: Provided by the patient's body weight and the therapist's thigh pressed against the patient.

Mobilization: The therapist's hands are on the ipsilateral area over the anterior thorax and on the contralateral posterior thorax during the overpressure.

Direction of Force: Therapist passively axially rotates the patient for an overpressure (right figure page 265).

Ask questions regarding the reproduction of symptoms while observing the quality and quantity of active movements. Assess the movements from the top down, noting segmental recruitment of motion. Identify deviations from the normal planes of motion including rotation, side bending, forward, or backward bending.

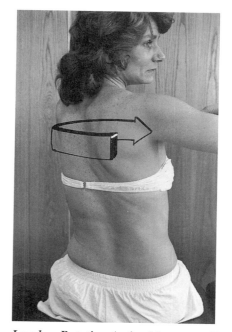 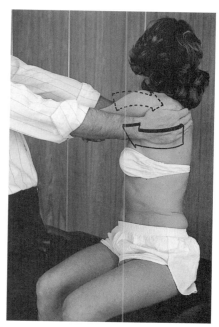

Lumbar Rotation Active Movement Testing and Overpressure

Lumbar (T11/12–L5/S1)

Passive Physiologic Segmental Movement Testing: Forward Bending

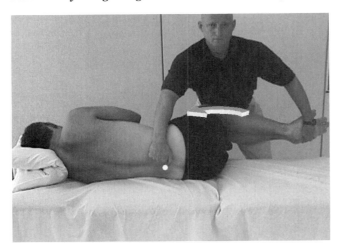

Patient Position: Patient is side lying near the edge of the table with trunk and pelvis in a neutral spinal posture.

Therapist Position: Therapist stands at the level of the lumbar spine facing the patient.

Stabilization: Therapist's proximal forearm and the patient's body weight stabilize the upper trunk in a neutral position.

Mobilization: Therapist flexes one or both legs of the patient, resting the patient's knees on the therapist's abdomen/groin area, while supporting the lower legs with the distal hand. Therapist palpates the interspinous space of the segment to be tested with the proximal hand.

Direction of Force: Therapist flexes the patient's hips and lumbar spine, and palpates for an increase in interspinous distance and a relative increase in soft tissue tension at this level.

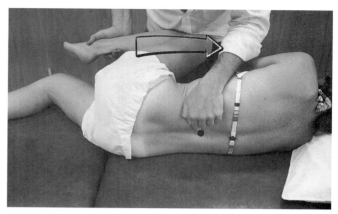

Passive Forward Bending Segmental Movement Testing with One Lower Extremity

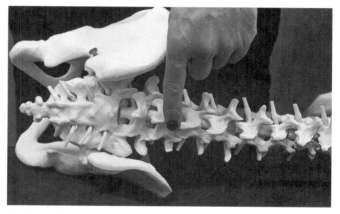

Skeletal Passive Forward Bending Segmental Movement Testing Palpation

Lumbar (T11/12–L5/S1)

Passive Physiologic Segmental Movement Testing: Backward Bending

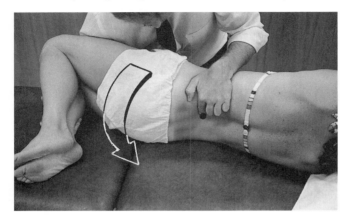

Patient Position: Patient is side-lying near the edge of the table with trunk and pelvis in a neutral spinal posture.

Therapist Position: Therapist stands at the level of the lumbar spine facing the patient.

Stabilization: Therapist's proximal arm and the patient's body weight stabilize the upper trunk in a neutral position.

Mobilization: Therapist extends one or both hips of the patient while supporting the lower leg(s) with the distal hand. Therapist palpates the interspinous space of the segment to be tested with the proximal hand.

Direction of Force: Therapist extends the patient's hips and lumbar spine and palpates for a decrease in interspinous distance and a relative decrease in soft tissue tension at this level.

Lumbar (T11/12-L5/S1)

Passive Physiologic Segmental Movement Testing: Side Bending

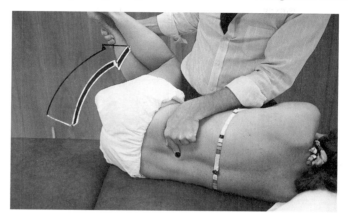

Patient Position: Patient is side-lying near the edge of the table with trunk and pelvis in a neutral spinal posture.

Therapist Position: Therapist stands at the level of the lumbar spine facing the patient.

Stabilization: Therapist's proximal forearm and the patient's body weight stabilize the upper trunk in a neutral position.

Mobilization: Therapist grasps the patient's distal legs near the ankle and flexes both the knees and the hips to less than 90°, supporting the patient's thighs on the therapist's thighs. Therapist palpates the ipsilateral aspect of the interspinous space of the segment to be tested with the proximal hand.

Direction of Force: Patient's legs are passively elevated (rotated) toward the therapist to produce a side bending motion in the lumbar spine. Therapist palpates for the distal palpable spinous process to move into the palpating finger, producing a decrease in the interspinous space and a relative decrease in soft tissue tension at this level (figure above).

Side bending to the opposite side can be accomplished from this same starting position. Therapist palpates on the inferior aspect of the interspinous space (bottom figure page 270) while lowering the flexed hip and knee complex to produce side bending in the lumbar spine in the opposite direction (top figure page 270).

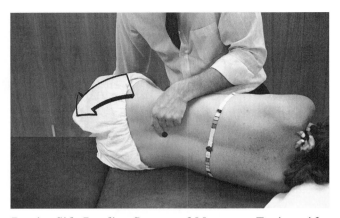

Passive Side Bending Segmental Movement Testing with Lower Extremity Lowering

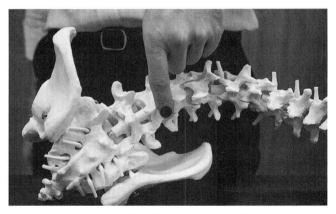

Skeletal Passive Side Bending Segmental Movement Testing

Lumbar (T11/12–L5/S1)

Passive Physiologic Segmental Movement Testing: Rotation

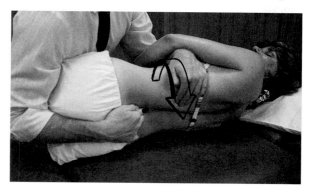

Patient Position: Patient is side-lying near the edge of the table with trunk and pelvis in a neutral position.

Therapist Position: Therapist stands at the level of the lumbar spine facing the patient.

Stabilization: Therapist's distal forearm and hand stabilize the pelvis in a neutral position.

Mobilization: Therapist's proximal forearm and hand rest on the patient's upper trunk while the distal hand palpates on the contralateral aspect of the appropriate interspinous space.

Direction of Force: Therapist passively rotates the patient's trunk posteriorly with the proximal forearm/hand while palpating for the superior spinous process to move into the palpating finger of the distal hand, as well as for an increase in soft tissue tension at this level.

Lumbar (T11/12–L5/S1)

Passive Accessory Movement Testing: Central Posterior-Anterior Pressure

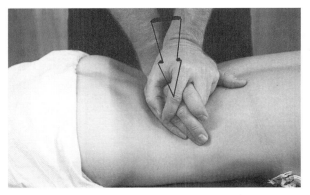

Patient Position: Patient lies prone near the edge of the table with the lumbar spine in a neutral position.

Therapist Position: Therapist stands lateral to the lumbar spine facing the table with shoulders positioned directly over the patient's lumbar area.

Stabilization: Provided by the patient's body weight.

Mobilization: Therapist's pisiform area of one hand (the dummy hand) is placed over the spinous process of the level to be assessed. The therapist's other hand (the mobilization hand) grasps the fingers of the dummy hand. The heel of the mobilization hand is placed over the pisiform area of the dummy hand. The therapist's arms are straight with the upper body, centered over the hands, and the shoulders adducted.

Direction of Force: Posterior to anterior pressure is applied through the spinous process of the level assessed.

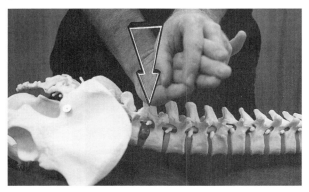

Skeletal Lumbar Central Posterior-Anterior Pressure

Lumbar (T11/12–L5/S1)

Passive Accessory Movement Testing: Unilateral Posterior-Anterior Pressure

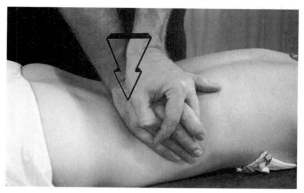

Patient Position: Patient lies prone near the edge of the table with the lumbar spine in a neutral position.

Therapist Position: Therapist stands lateral to the lumbar spine facing the table with his/her shoulders positioned directly over the patient's lumbar area.

Stabilization: Provided by the patient's body weight.

Mobilization: Therapist's pisiform area of one hand (the dummy hand) is placed over the contralateral transverse process of the level to be assessed. The therapist's other hand (the mobilization hand) grasps the fingers of the dummy hand. The heel of the mobilization hand is placed over the pisiform area of the dummy hand. The therapist's arms are straight with the upper body, centered over the hands, and the shoulders adducted.

Direction of Force: Posterior to anterior pressure is applied through the transverse process at the level assessed.

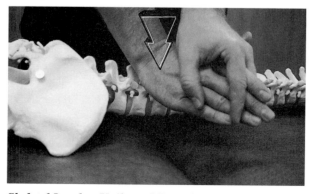

Skeletal Lumbar Unilateral Posterior-Anterior Pressure

Lumbar (T11/12–L5/S1)

Passive Accessory Movement Testing: Transverse Pressure

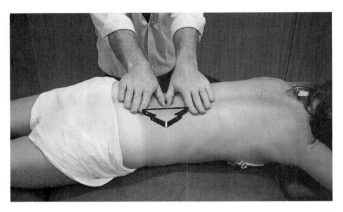

Patient Position: Patient lies prone near the edge of the table with the lumbar spine in a neutral position.

Therapist Position: Therapist stands lateral to the lumbar spine facing the table with the therapist's arms parallel to the plane of the patient's trunk.

Stabilization: Provided by the patient's body weight.

Mobilization: Therapist's thumbs are placed together along the ipsilateral side of the spinous process at the level to be assessed with the remainder of the hands/fingers relaxed. Elbows are straight and the upper extremities are maintained horizontal to the plane of the patient's back.

Direction of Force: Pressure through the side of the spinous process is directed toward the contralateral side in a transverse direction.

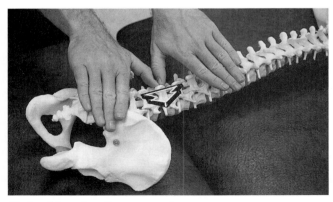

Skeletal Lumbar Transverse Pressure

Lumbar (T11/12–L5/S1)

Passive Accessory Movement Testing: Dorsal Glide

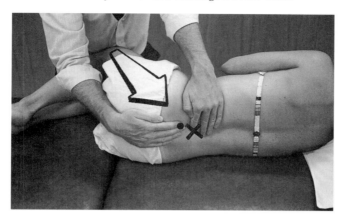

This is a special test for instability.

Patient Position: Patient is side-lying near the edge of the table with the trunk and pelvis in a neutral position and the hips flexed to less than 90°.

Therapist Position: Therapist stands directly opposite to the patient's flexed hips/knees facing the lumbar spine.

Stabilization: Patient's body weight and the therapist's cephalic hand stabilize the superior segment.

Mobilization: Therapist's caudal hand palpates the appropriate interspinous space.

Direction of Force: Therapist imparts a dorsal glide of the lower partner of the motion segment to be tested by pushing against the patient's distal femurs in a posterior direction. The caudal hand is placed over the dorsum of the sacrum. Therapist's caudal hand assists the return of the sacrum and the associated lumbar levels to the neutral starting position.

Minimal dorsal movement normally occurs with this test unless instability of the associated level exists.

Thoracic (T3/4–T10/11)

Active Movement Testing

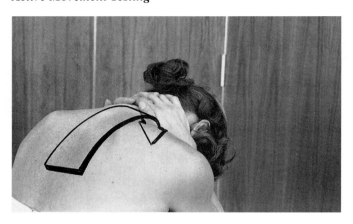

Observe the patient standing or sitting from an anterior, a posterior, and both lateral views. Note any asymmetries using major landmarks and differences in the two positions.

Patient Position: Patient sits in neutral posture. Placement of the upper extremities can vary from crossed behind the neck (figure above and all figures page 277), to crossed in the "genie position," to crossed over the chest.

Therapist Position: Stand and observe the patient's movement.

Stabilization: Provided by the patient's body weight.

Mobilization: Patient moves actively through thoracic forward bending (figure above), backward bending (top figure page 277), side bending (middle figure page 277), and rotation movements (bottom figure page 277).

Direction of Force: Forward bending, backward bending, side bending, and rotation.

Ask questions regarding the reproduction of symptoms while observing the quality and quantity of active movements. Assess the movements from the top down, noting segmental recruitment of motion. Identify deviations from the normal planes of motion including rotation, side bending, forward, or backward bending.

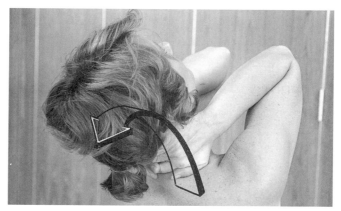

Thoracic Backward Bending Active Movement Testing

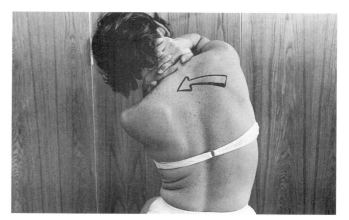

Thoracic Side Bending Active Movement Testing

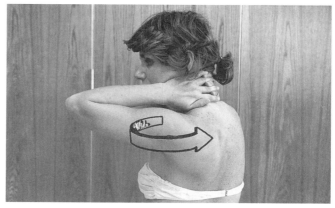

Thoracic Rotation Active Movement Testing

Thoracic (T3/4–T10/11)

**Passive Physiologic Segmental Movement Testing: Forward Bending
(Weight Bearing)**

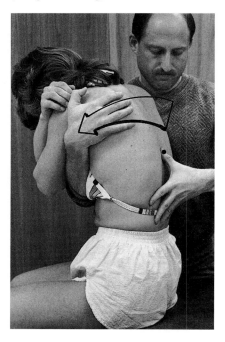

Patient Position: Patient sits with lower extremities supported and the lumbar spine in a neutral position with arms crossed behind the head, or at the shoulders, with the head/neck relaxed.

Therapist Position: Therapist stands alongside the patient.

Stabilization: Therapist's body and arm supporting the patient provide stabilization.

Mobilization: Therapist cradles the patient's upper extremities under bilateral axillae. Patient's opposite shoulder or scapular area is supported to facilitate movement. Therapist's other hand palpates between the spinous processes.

Direction of Force: Therapist flexes the patient's trunk in an increasing arc of motion as movement is assessed from T3 to T10. Therapist notes gapping of the spinous processes or increased soft tissue tension at this level.

Thoracic (T3/4–T10/11)

Passive Physiologic Segmental Movement Testing: Backward Bending (Weight Bearing)

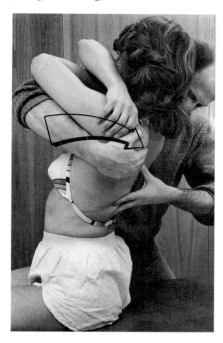

Patient Position: Patient sits with lower extremities supported and the lumbar spine in a neutral position with arms crossed behind the head, or at the shoulders, with the head/neck relaxed.

Therapist Position: Therapist stands alongside the patient.

Stabilization: Therapist's body and arm supporting the patient provide stabilization.

Mobilization: Therapist cradles the patient's upper extremities under bilateral axillae. Patient's opposite shoulder or scapular area is supported to facilitate movement.

Direction of Force: Therapist extends the patient's trunk in an increasing arc of motion as movement is assessed from T3 to T10. The upper thoracic levels require additional shoulder flexion movement of the crossed arms to produce thoracic extension. Therapist palpates between spinous processes to note approximation of the spinous processes or decreased soft tissue tension at this level.

Thoracic (T3/4–T10/11)

Passive Physiologic Segmental Movement Testing: Side Bending (Weight Bearing)

Patient Position: Patient sits with lower extremities supported and the lumbar spine in a neutral position with arms crossed behind the head, or at the shoulders (both figures page 281), with the head/neck relaxed.

Therapist Position: Therapist stands alongside the patient.

Stabilization: Therapist's body and arm supporting the patient provide stabilization.

Mobilization: Therapist cradles the patient's upper extremities under bilateral axillae to side bend the patient away from the therapist (left figure page 281). To side bend the patient toward the therapist, the therapist hooks through the patient's closest arm to grasp under the opposite axilla (right figure page 281). Patient's opposite shoulder or scapular area is supported to facilitate movement. Therapist palpates between spinous processes on the concave side of the curve.

Direction of Force: Therapist side bends the patient's trunk away from the therapist in an increasing arc of motion as movement is assessed from T3 to T10 by a lifting force with the body under the closest shoulder while assisting the opposite shoulder to drop (left figure page 281). Therapist side bends the trunk toward the therapist in an increasing arc of motion as movement is assessed from T3 to T10 by lifting the opposite shoulder and assisting downward movement of the patient's trunk on the side next to the therapist (right figure page 281). Therapist palpates approximation of the spinous processes or a decrease in soft tissue tension at this level.

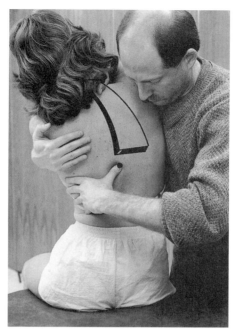 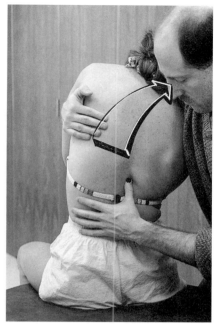

Passive Physiologic Segmental Movement Testing:

Side Bending Away   *Side Bending Toward*

Thoracic (T3/4–T10/11)

Passive Physiologic Segmental Movement Testing: Rotation (Weight Bearing)

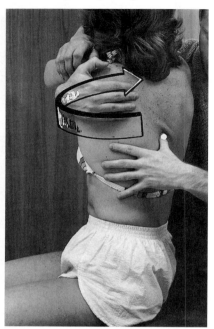

Patient Position: Patient sits with lower extremities supported and the lumbar spine in a neutral position with the arms crossed behind the head, or at the shoulders, with the head/neck relaxed.

Therapist Position: Therapist stands alongside the patient.

Stabilization: Therapist's body and arm supporting the patient provide stabilization.

Mobilization: Therapist cradles the patient's upper extremities under bilateral axillae. Patient's opposite shoulder or scapular area is supported to facilitate movement.

Direction of Force: Therapist axially rotates the patient's trunk toward the therapist in an increasing arc of motion as movement is assessed from T3 to T10 by pulling at the opposite shoulder and pushing with the trunk on the side next to the patient. Therapist palpates on the concave side of the curve between spinous processes to note the movement of the upper spinous process on the lower spinous process or increased soft tissue tension at this level.

Thoracic (T3/4–T10/11)

Passive Physiologic Segmental Movement Testing: Forward Bending (Nonweight Bearing)

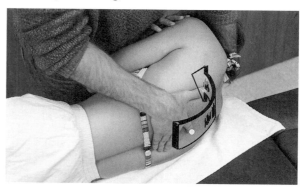

Patient Position: Patient is side-lying with the lumbar spine in a neutral position and hands clasped behind neck or arms crossed holding shoulders.

Therapist Position: Therapist faces the patient.

Stabilization: Therapist's trunk and upper extremity stabilize the patient's position.

Mobilization: While supporting the patient's upper trunk off the table by cradling the patient's neck and upper extremities and resting the upper extremities in the therapist's hip flexor crease area, the therapist's caudal hand palpates between the spinous processes of the segment to be assessed.

Direction of Force: Therapist flexes the patient's thoracic spine in an increasing arc of motion from T3 to T10. Therapist palpates a gapping of the superior spinous process on the inferior spinous process or an increase in soft tissue tension at this level.

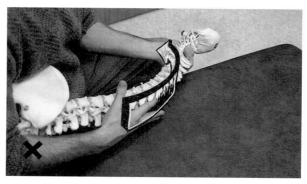

Skeletal Passive Foreward Bending Segmental Movement Testing

Thoracic (T3/4–T10/11)

Passive Physiologic Segmental Movement Testing: Backward Bending (Nonweight Bearing)

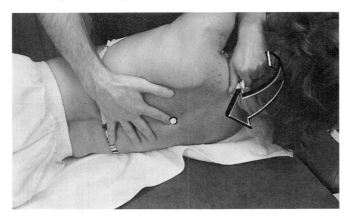

Patient Position: Patient is side-lying with the lumbar spine in a neutral position and hands clasped behind neck or arms crossed holding shoulders.

Therapist Position: Therapist faces the patient.

Stabilization: Therapist's trunk and upper extremity stabilize the patient's position.

Mobilization: While supporting the patient's upper trunk off the table by cradling the patient's neck and upper extremities and resting the upper extremities in the therapist's hip flexor crease area, the therapist's caudal hand palpates between spinous processes of the segment to be assessed.

Direction of Force: Therapist extends the patient's thoracic spine in an increasing arc of motion from T3 to T10. Therapist palpates between spinous processes to note approximation of the spinous processes or decreased soft tissue tension at this level.

Thoracic (T3/4–T10/11)

Passive Physiologic Segmental Movement Testing: Side Bending (Nonweight Bearing)

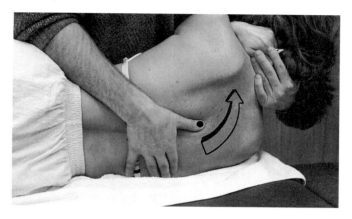

Patient Position: Patient is side-lying with the lumbar spine in a neutral position and hands clasped behind neck (figure above) or arms crossed holding the shoulders. Patient either rests on the table or with the upper thorax off the table.

Therapist Position: Therapist faces the patient.

Stabilization: Therapist's trunk and upper extremity stabilize the patient's position.

Mobilization: While supporting the patient's upper trunk by cradling the patient's neck and upper extremities, the therapist's caudal hand palpates between spinous processes of the segment assessed on the concave side of the curve.

Direction of Force: Therapist side bends the patient's thoracic spine in an increasing arc of motion from T3 to T10 by lifting the patient off the table (figure above) or with the upper thorax off the table by side bending toward the floor (bottom figure page 286). Therapist notes approximation of spinous processes or decreased soft tissue tension at this level.

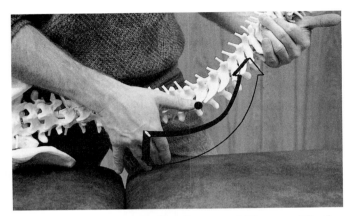

Skeletal Passive Side Bending Segmental Movement Testing

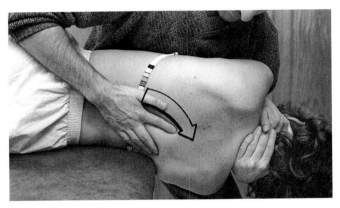

Passive Side Bending Away Segmental
Movement Testing

Thoracic (T3/4–T10/11)

Passive Physiologic Segmental Movement Testing: Rotation (Nonweight Bearing)

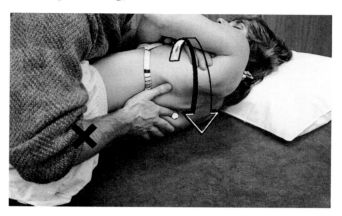

Patient Position: Patient is side-lying with the lumbar spine in a neutral position and the head turned in the direction of rotation.

Therapist Position: Therapist faces the patient.

Stabilization: Therapist's body and caudal forearm provide stabilization along the lumbar spine/pelvis.

Mobilization: Therapist's cephalic hand is placed across the patient's anterior chest wall (figure above) or at the shoulder (top figure page 288). The caudal hand palpates between spinous processes of the segment on the lower (opposite) side.

Direction of Force: Therapist axially rotates the patient's thoracic spine in an increasing arc of motion from T3 to T10 with the cephalic hand at the shoulder or thorax. Therapist notes the spinous process of the level above moving into the finger/thumb or increased soft tissue tension at this level.

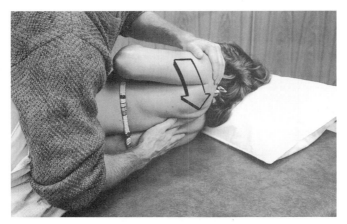

Passive Rotation Segmental Movement Testing
at Shoulder

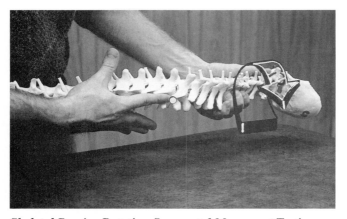

Skeletal Passive Rotation Segmental Movement Testing

Thoracic (T3/4–T10/11)

Passive Accessory Movement Testing: Central Posterior-Anterior Pressure

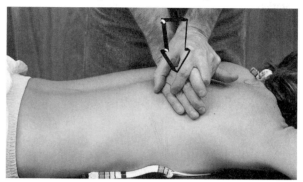

Patient Position: Patient lies prone with the cervical and lumbar spine in neutral alignment.

Therapist Position: Therapist stands alongside and facing the patient.

Stabilization: Provided by the patient's body weight.

Mobilization: Therapist's pisiform area of one hand (the dummy hand) is placed over the spinous process of the level to be assessed. The therapist's other hand (the mobilization hand) grasps the fingers of the dummy hand. The heel of the mobilization hand is placed over the pisiform area of the dummy hand. The therapist's arms are straight with the upper body, centered over the hands, and the shoulders adducted.

Direction of Force: Posterior to anterior pressure is applied through the spinous process of the level assessed.

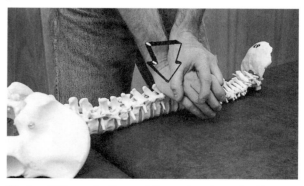

Skeletal Thoracic Central Posterior-Anterior Pressure

Thoracic (T3/4–T10/11)

Passive Accessory Movement Testing: Unilateral Posterior-Anterior Pressure

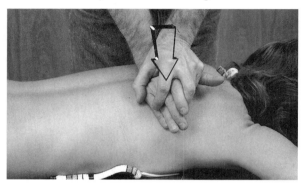

Patient Position: Patient lies prone with the cervical and lumbar spine in neutral alignment.

Therapist Position: Therapist stands on the side opposite to be mobilized facing the patient.

Stabilization: Provided by the patient's body weight.

Mobilization: Therapist's pisiform area of one hand (the dummy hand) is placed over the contralateral transverse process of the level to be assessed. The therapist's other hand (the mobilization hand) grasps the fingers of the dummy hand. The heel of the mobilization hand is placed over the pisiform area of the dummy hand. The therapist's arms are straight with the upper body, centered over the hands, and the shoulders adducted.

Direction of Force: Posterior to anterior pressure is applied through the transverse process at the level assessed.

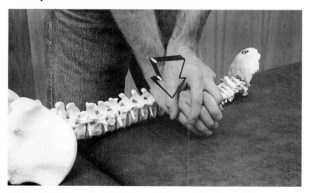

Skeletal Thoracic Unilateral Posterior-Anterior Pressure

Thoracic (T3/4–T10/11)

Passive Accessory Movement Testing: Transverse Pressure

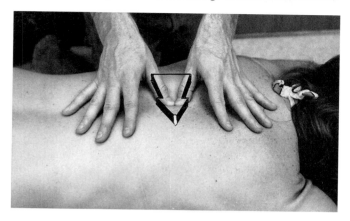

Patient Position: Patient lies prone with the cervical and lumbar spine in neutral alignment.

Therapist Position: Therapist stands alongside and facing the patient.

Stabilization: Provided by the patient's body weight.

Mobilization: Therapist's thumbs are placed together alongside the spinous process at the level to be assessed with the remainder of the hands/fingers relaxed. Elbows are straight and the upper extremities are maintained horizontal to the plane of the patient's back.

Direction of Force: Pressure through the side of the spinous process is directed toward the contralateral side in a transverse direction.

Thoracic (T3/4–T10/11)

Passive Accessory Movement Testing: Bilateral Posterior-Anterior Pressure

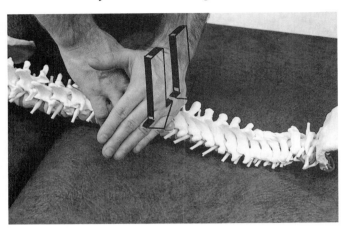

Patient Position: Patient lies prone with the cervical and lumbar spine in neutral alignment.

Therapist Position: Therapist stands alongside and facing the patient.

Stabilization: Provided by the patient's body weight.

Mobilization: Therapist's index and middle fingers of the caudal hand (the dummy hand) are placed on the transverse processes of the level to be assessed with the remainder of the hand relaxed (top and middle figures page 293). The hypothenar eminence of the cephalic hand is placed over the index and middle fingers of the dummy hand (figure above and bottom figure page 293).

Direction of Force: Posterior to anterior pressure is applied to the transverse processes by the cephalic hand (figure above).

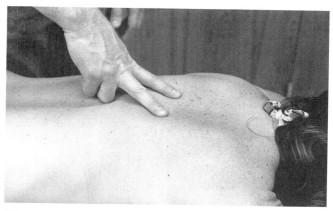

Thoracic Bilateral Posterior-Anterior Pressure
Dummy Hand Positioning

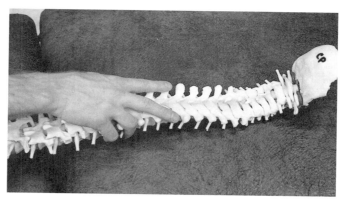

Skeletal Thoracic Bilateral Posterior-Anterior Pressure
Dummy Hand Positioning

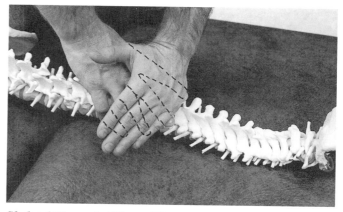

Skeletal Thoracic Bilateral Posterior-Anterior Pressure
Hypothenar Eminence Positioning

Thoracic (T2–T12)

Passive Accessory Movement Testing: Rib Posterior-Anterior Pressure

Patient Position: Patient lies prone with the upper extremity position variable (in the small of the back for the upper ribs).

Therapist Position: Therapist stands on the contralateral side facing the patient at the level to be assessed.

Stabilization: The contralateral transverse process and lamina of the rib to be mobilized are stabilized with the heel of one hand.

Mobilization: The pisiform area of the second hand is placed over the posterior angle of the rib to be mobilized with the remainder of the hand relaxed.

Direction of Force: The upper ribs are mobilized in an anterior, lateral, and inferior direction. The middle ribs are mobilized in an anterior and lateral direction. The lower ribs are mobilized in an anterior, lateral, and superior direction.

Upper Rib Technique:

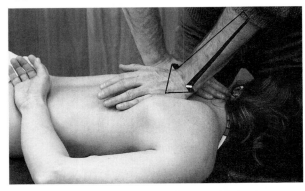

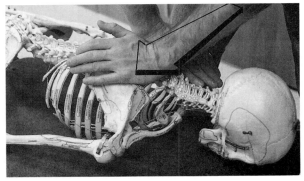

Skeletal Upper Rib Posterior-Anterior Pressure

Middle Rib Technique:

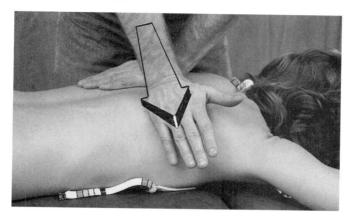

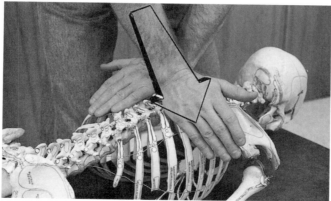

Skeletal Middle Rib Posterior-Anterior Pressure

Lower Rib Technique:

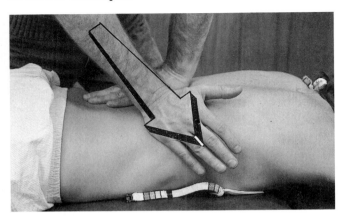

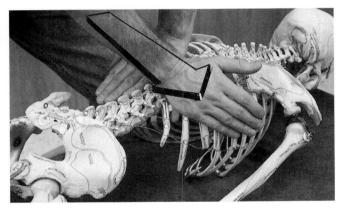

Skeletal Lower Rib Posterior-Anterior Pressure

Cervical

Active Movement Testing/Overpressure: Forward Bending

Observe the patient standing and sitting from an anterior, a posterior, and both lateral views. Note any asymmetries using major landmarks and differences in the two positions.

Patient Position: Patient sits with the feet supported.

Therapist Position: Therapist stands to the side of the patient.

Stabilization: One hand is placed centrally over the patient's upper thoracic spine during the overpressure.

Mobilization: The other hand and forearm is placed over the top of the patient's head from the occiput to the forehead during the overpressure.

Direction of Force: After observing active movement (left figure page 298), the therapist's mobilizing hand and forearm impart a force pulling the head forward flexing the neck in the direction of the stabilization hand to bow the cervical spine (right figure page 298).

Ask questions regarding the reproduction of symptoms while observing the quality and quantity of active movements. Assess the movements from the top down, noting segmental recruitment of motion. Identify deviations from the normal planes of motion including rotation, side bending, forward, or backward bending.

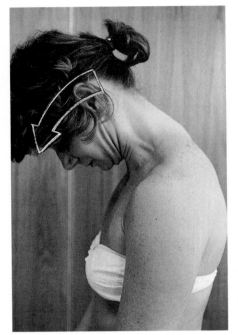 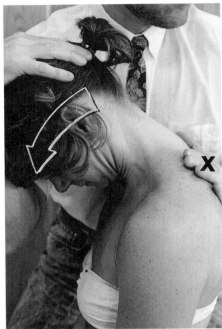

Forward Bending Active Movement Testing and Overpressure

Cervical

Active Movement Testing/Overpressure: Backward Bending

Observe the patient standing and sitting from an anterior, a posterior, and both lateral views. Note any asymmetries using major landmarks and differences in the two positions.

Patient Position: Patient sits with the feet supported.

Therapist Position: Therapist stands to the side of the patient.

Stabilization: One hand is placed over the sternum anteriorly during the overpressure.

Mobilization: The other hand and forearm is placed over the anterior superior portion of the head during the overpressure.

Direction of Force: After observing active movement (left figure page 300), the therapist's mobilizing hand and forearm impart a force pulling the head backward extending the neck in the direction of the stabilization hand to bow the cervical spine (right figure page 300).

Ask questions regarding the reproduction of symptoms while observing the quality and quantity of active movements. Assess the movements from the top down, noting segmental recruitment of motion. Identify deviations from the normal planes of motion including rotation, side bending, forward, or backward bending.

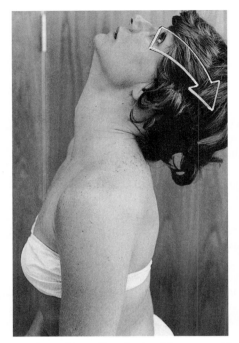 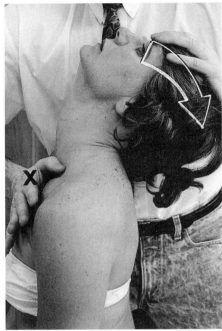

Backward Bending Active Movement Testing and Overpressure

Cervical

Active Movement Testing/Overpressure: Side Bending

Observe the patient standing and sitting from an anterior, a posterior, and both lateral views. Note any asymmetries using major landmarks and differences in the two positions.

Patient Position: Patient sits with the feet supported.

Therapist Position: Therapist stands behind the patient.

Stabilization: For the overpressure: Technique A: The left hand is placed under the axilla on the left supporting the upper thorax. Technique B: The right hand is placed over the shoulder girdle on the right.

Mobilization: For the overpressure: Technique A: The right hand and forearm is placed along the right side of the patient's neck and head. Technique B: The left hand and forearm is placed over the right side of the patient's neck and head.

Direction of Force: After observing active movement (top figure page 302), the therapist imparts a force pulling the neck/head further to the left side bending the left side to bow the cervical spine in both techniques. This technique is repeated in the same way to the right. Technique A should have more motion and a harder capsular end-feel. Technique B should be more limited with a soft tissue/muscular end-feel.

Ask questions regarding the reproduction of symptoms while observing the quality and quantity of active movements. Assess the movements from the top down, noting segmental recruitment of motion. Identify deviations from the normal planes of motion including rotation, side bending, forward, or backward bending.

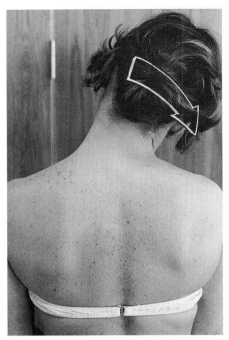

Side Bending Active Movement Testing

Technique A: *Technique B:*

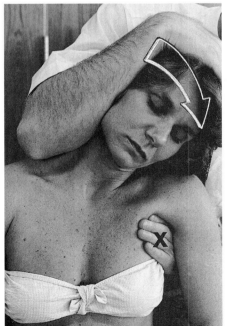   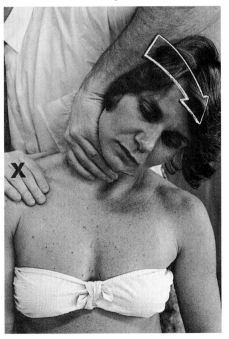

Side Bending Overpressures

Cervical

Active Movement Testing/Overpressure: Rotation

Observe the patient standing and sitting from an anterior, a posterior, and both lateral views. Note any asymmetries using major landmarks and differences in the two positions.

Patient Position: Patient sits with the feet supported.

Therapist Position: Therapist stands behind the patient.

Stabilization: Stabilization is provided by the therapist's trunk from behind and from the left upper arm placed over the patient's left shoulder anteriorly during the overpressure.

Mobilization: The therapist's right hand is placed over the left side of the patient's head with the therapist's left hand placed over the right side of the patient's head during the overpressure.

Direction of Force: After observing active movement (left figure page 304), the therapist produces axial rotation by pulling the patient's head around to the right with both hands (right figure page 304). This technique is repeated to the left.

Ask questions regarding the reproduction of symptoms while observing the quality and quantity of active movements. Assess the movements from the top down, noting segmental recruitment of motion. Identify deviations from the normal planes of motion including rotation, side bending, forward, or backward bending.

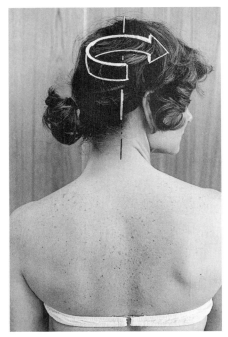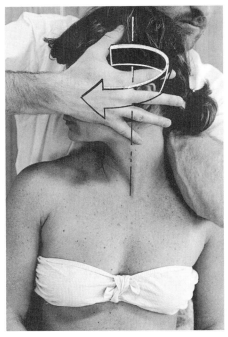

Rotation Active Movement Testing and Overpressure

Cervical

General Passive Physiologic Movement Testing:
Forward Bending/Side Bending/Backward Bending

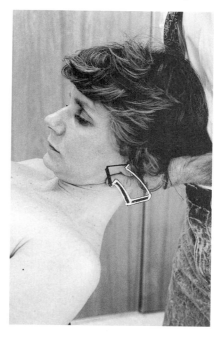

Patient Position: Patient lies supine with the head/neck off the edge of the table in a neutral resting position.

Therapist Position: Therapist stands or sits at the head of the patient.

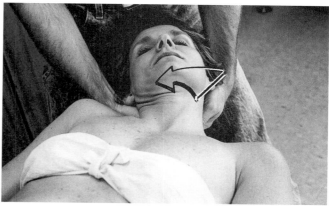

Stabilization: Provided by the patient's body weight.

Mobilization: Therapist places both hands on the patient's occiput.

Direction of Force: Therapist slowly moves the head/neck through the full range of forward bending (top figure page 305), side bending (bottom figure page 305), or backward bending (figure below).

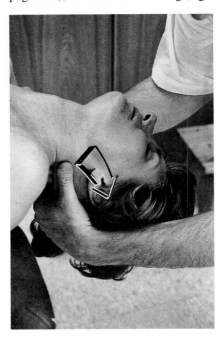

Cervical

General Passive Physiologic Movement Testing: Rotation

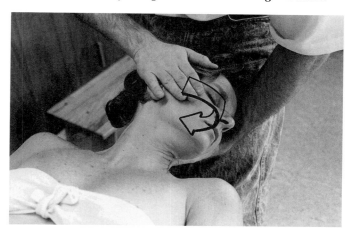

Patient Position: Patient lies supine with the head/neck off the edge of the table in a neutral resting position.

Therapist Position: Therapist stands or sits at the head of the patient.

Stabilization: Provided by the patient's body weight.

Mobilization: Therapist places a hand on each side of the patient's head.

Direction of Force: Therapist slowly moves the head through the full range of rotation.

Cervical

Axial Compression Testing

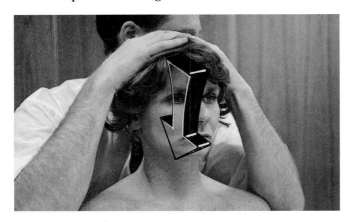

Patient Position: Patient sits with the feet supported.

Therapist Position: Therapist stands behind the patient.

Stabilization: Therapist's trunk supports from behind while the therapist's elbows support at the shoulders.

Mobilization: Therapist places both hands on top of the patient's head.

Direction of Force: Therapist slowly imparts a downward force compressing the cervical spine. This is held for 3 to 5 seconds and released slowly. It is important to not allow movement of the head/neck during this test.

Indications: Reproduction of symptoms makes this a positive test for weight bearing structures. Occasionally, this test also alleviates symptoms.

Cervical

Axial Decompression Testing (Traction)

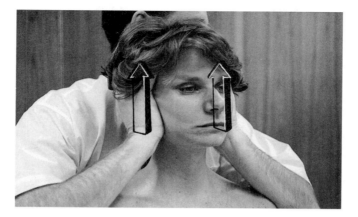

Patient Position: Patient sits with the feet supported.

Therapist Position: Therapist stands behind the patient.

Stabilization: Therapist's trunk supports from behind while the therapist's elbows support on top of the shoulders.

Mobilization: Therapist places the heel of both hands over the base of the occiput, including the mastoid processes bilaterally. Fingers of both hands support the lateral sides of the head.

Direction of Force: Therapist lifts cephalically with both hands while adducting the elbows and forcing the shoulders downward.

Indications: A change in symptoms makes this a positive test for weight bearing or ligamentous structures.

Cervical

General Quadrant Position Testing

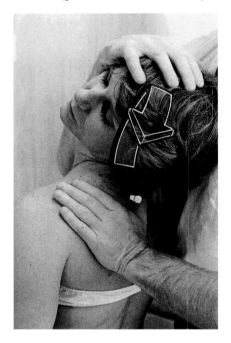

This is a special test for the vertebral artery (see page 337).

Patient Position: Patient sits with the feet supported.

Therapist Position: Therapist stands behind the patient.

Stabilization: Therapist's left hand is placed over the left side of the patient's upper thoracic spine.

Mobilization: Therapist's right hand and forearm is placed over the right side of the patient's neck and head.

Direction of Force: Therapist assists the patient in performing left rotation, left side bending, and backward bending simultaneously. If there is no reproduction of symptoms through the passive range, the therapist applies a passive overpressure with the right hand and forearm in the direction of the movement. This technique is also repeated to the right side.

Cervical-Thoracic Junction (C7/T1–T2/3)

Passive Physiologic Movement Testing: Forward Bending (Weight Bearing)

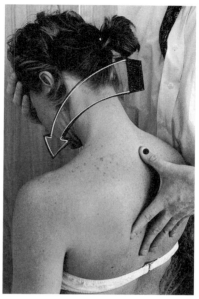

Patient Position: Patient sits in a neutral cervical-thoracic spinal posture.

Therapist Position: Therapist stands alongside facing the patient.

Stabilization: Therapist's body provides stabilization.

Mobilization: Therapist's anterior hand is placed over the front of the patient's head or the head/neck is cradled by the therapist's upper extremity.

Direction of Force: Therapist flexes the cervical-thoracic spine while palpating between spinous processes for an increase in soft tissue tension or a gapping of the spinous processes at the level assessed.

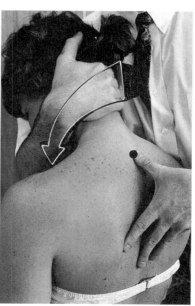

Cervical-Thoracic Junction (C7/T1–T2/3)

Passive Physiologic Segmental Movement Testing: Backward Bending (Weight Bearing)

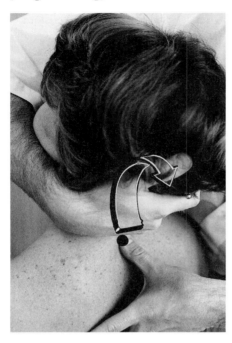

Patient Position: Patient sits in a neutral cervical-thoracic spinal posture.

Therapist Position: Therapist stands alongside facing the patient.

Stabilization: Therapist's body provides stabilization.

Mobilization: Therapist's anterior hand is placed over the back of the patient's head or the head/neck is cradled by the therapist's upper extremity.

Direction of Force: Therapist backward bends the cervical-thoracic spine while palpating between spinous processes for a decrease in soft tissue tension or an approximation of the spinous processes at the level assessed.

Cervical-Thoracic Junction (C7/T1–T2/3)

Passive Physiologic Segmental Movement Testing: Side Bending (Weight Bearing)

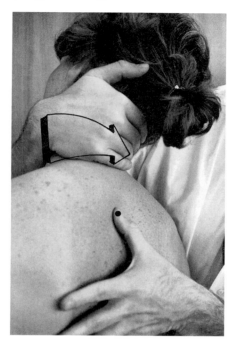

Patient Position: Patient sits in a neutral cervical-thoracic spinal posture.

Therapist Position: Therapist stands alongside facing the patient.

Stabilization: Therapist's body provides stabilization.

Mobilization: Therapist's anterior hand grasps the opposite side of the patient's head or the head/neck is cradled by the therapist's upper extremity.

Direction of Force: Therapist side bends the cervical-thoracic spine away from or toward the therapist while palpating between spinous processes on the concave side of the curve for a decrease in soft tissue tension or an approximation of the spinous processes at the level assessed.

Cervical-Thoracic Junction (C7/T1–T2/3)

Passive Physiologic Segmental Movement Testing: Rotation (Weight Bearing)

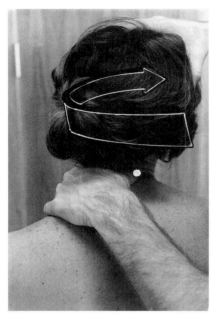

Patient Position: Patient sits in a neutral cervical-thoracic spinal posture.

Therapist Position: Therapist stands alongside facing the patient.

Stabilization: Therapist's body provides stabilization.

Mobilization: Therapist's anterior hand is placed on top of the patient's head or the head/neck is cradled by the therapist's upper extremity. Therapist also supports the ipsilateral side of the patient's head with the therapist's trunk.

Direction of Force: Therapist axially rotates the cervical-thoracic spine toward the therapist while palpating between spinous processes on the convex side of the curve for an increase in soft tissue tension or movement of the superior spinous process into the palpating finger at the level assessed.

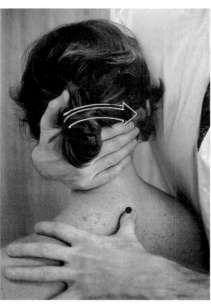

Cervical-Thoracic Junction (C7/T1–T2/3)

Passive Physiologic Segmental Movement Testing: Forward Bending (Nonweight Bearing)

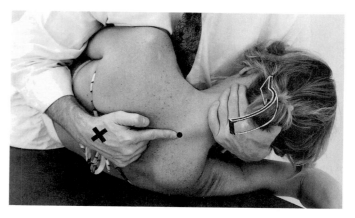

Patient Position: Patient is side-lying in a neutral cervical-thoracic spinal posture.

Therapist Position: Therapist faces the patient.

Stabilization: Therapist's trunk and upper extremities stabilize the patient's position.

Mobilization: Therapist's cephalic hand/forearm cradles the patient's head/neck.

Direction of Force: Therapist flexes the cervical-thoracic spine while palpating with the caudal hand between spinous processes for an increase in soft tissue tension or a gapping of the spinous processes at the level assessed.

Cervical-Thoracic Junction (C7/T1–T2/3)

Passive Physiologic Segmental Movement Testing: Backward Bending (Nonweight Bearing)

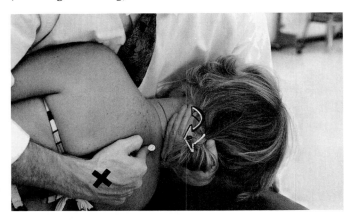

Patient Position: Patient is side-lying in a neutral cervical-thoracic spinal posture.

Therapist Position: Therapist faces the patient.

Stabilization: Therapist's trunk and upper extremities stabilize the patient's position.

Mobilization: Therapist's cephalic hand/forearm cradles the patient's head/neck.

Direction of Force: Therapist backward bends the cervical-thoracic spine while palpating with the caudal hand between spinous processes for a decrease in soft tissue tension or an approximation of the spinous processes at the level assessed.

Cervical-Thoracic Junction (C7/T1–T2/3)

Passive Physiologic Segmental Movement Testing: Side Bending (Nonweight Bearing)

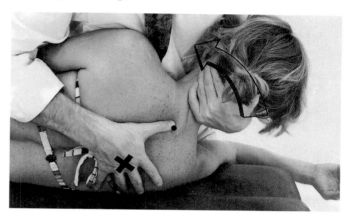

Patient Position: Patient is side-lying in a neutral cervical-thoracic spinal posture.

Therapist Position: Therapist faces the patient.

Stabilization: Therapist's trunk and upper extremities stabilize the patient's position.

Mobilization: Therapist's cephalic hand/forearm cradles the patient's head/neck.

Direction of Force: Therapist side bends the cervical-thoracic spine toward the therapist while palpating with the caudal hand between spinous processes on the concave side of the curve for a decrease in soft tissue tension or an approximation of the spinous processes at the level assessed.

Cervical-Thoracic Junction (C7/T1–T2/3)

Passive Physiologic Segmental Movement Testing: Rotation (Nonweight Bearing)

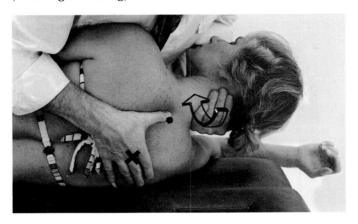

Patient Position: Patient is side-lying in a neutral cervical-thoracic spinal posture.

Therapist Position: Therapist faces the patient.

Stabilization: Therapist's trunk and upper extremities stabilize the patient's position.

Mobilization: Therapist's cephalic hand/forearm cradles the patient's head/neck.

Direction of Force: Therapist axially rotates the cervical-thoracic spine toward the therapist while palpating with the caudal hand between spinous processes on the convex side of the curve for an increase in soft tissue tension or movement of the superior spinous process into the palpating finger at the level assessed.

Cervical-Thoracic Junction (C7/T1–T2/3)

Passive Accessory Movement Testing: Dorsal Glide (Weight Bearing)

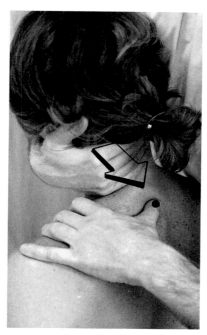

Patient Position: Patient sits in a neutral cervical-thoracic spinal posture.

Therapist Position: Therapist stands alongside facing the patient.

Stabilization: Therapist's body provides stabilization.

Mobilization: Therapist's anterior hand is placed over the patient's occiput with the upper arm at the forehead and the elbow at the front of the mandible.

Direction of Force: Therapist glides the head dorsally (patient may need to actively assist the therapist) while palpating between spinous processes for dorsal movement of the superior spinous process relative to the inferior spinous process at the level assessed.

Cervical-Thoracic Junction (C7/T1–T2/3)

Passive Accessory Movement Testing: Dorsal Glide (Nonweight Bearing)

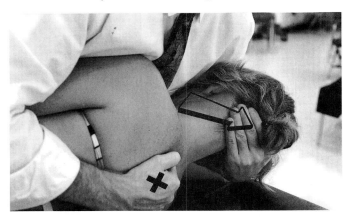

Patient Position: Patient is side-lying in a neutral cervical-thoracic spinal posture.

Therapist Position: Therapist faces the patient.

Stabilization: Therapist's trunk and upper extremities stabilize the patient's position.

Mobilization: Therapist's cephalic hand/forearm cradles the patient's head/neck.

Direction of Force: Therapist glides the head dorsally (patient may need to actively assist the therapist) while palpating with the caudal hand between spinous processes for dorsal movement of the superior spinous process relative to the inferior spinous process at the level assessed.

Cervical-Thoracic Junction (C7/T1–T2/3)

Passive Accessory Movement Testing: Central Posterior-Anterior Pressure

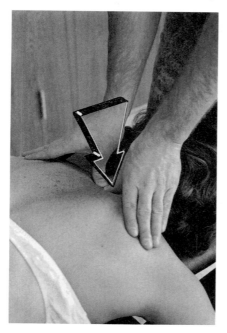

Patient Position: Patient lies prone with the spine in a neutral position.

Therapist Position: Therapist stands at the patient's head facing the patient.

Stabilization: Provided by the patient's body weight.

Mobilization: Therapist stands directly over the patient and places both thumb tips onto the spinous process of the level to be assessed.

Direction of Force: Therapist produces a posterior to anterior pressure on the spinous process.

Cervical-Thoracic Junction (C7/T1–T2/3)

Passive Accessory Movement Testing: Unilateral Posterior-Anterior Pressure

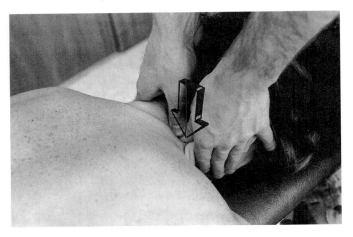

Patient Position: Patient lies prone with the spine in a neutral position.

Therapist Position: Therapist stands above the patient facing the patient's feet.

Stabilization: Provided by the patient's body weight.

Mobilization: The pads of the therapist's thumbs are placed over the posterior arch of the level to be assessed.

Direction of Force: Therapist moves the articular process in a posterior to anterior direction.

Cervical-Thoracic Junction (C7/T1–T2/3)

Passive Accessory Movement Testing: Transverse Pressure

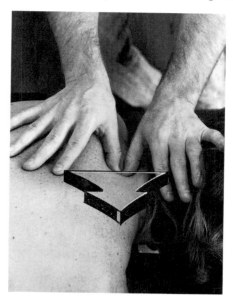

Patient Position: Patient lies prone with the spine in a neutral position.

Therapist Position: Therapist stands alongside facing the patient.

Stabilization: Provided by the patient's body weight.

Mobilization: The pads of the therapist's thumbs are placed on the ipsilateral side of the spinous process at the level to be assessed.

Direction of Force: Therapist moves the spinous process in a transverse direction.

Cervical-Thoracic Junction (C7/T1–T2/3)

Passive Accessory Movement Testing: First Rib (Sitting)

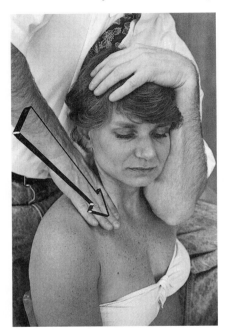

Patient Position: Patient sits.

Therapist Position: Therapist stands behind the patient.

Stabilization: Therapist's forearm cradles the contralateral side of the patient's head and neck with the hand that rests on the vertex of the patient's head. The therapist supports the patient's shoulder girdle with the therapist's leg on the opposite side to the rib mobilization.

Mobilization: Patient's head and neck are side bent slightly toward the side to be tested. The patient's head is rotated toward the side to be mobilized so that the T1 segment just begins to move. The lateral side of the therapist's index finger (distal to the metacarpophalangeal joint) is placed over the angle of the first rib with the therapist's forearm positioned in the direction of the movement.

Direction of Force: Therapist produces an anterior, inferior, and medial glide of the first rib.

Cervical-Thoracic Junction (C7/T1–T2/3)

Passive Accessory Movement Testing: First Rib (Supine)

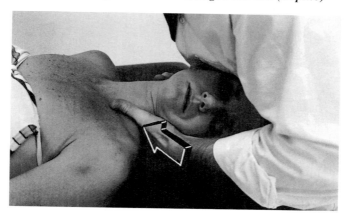

Patient Position: Patient lies supine.

Therapist Position: Therapist stands above the patient facing the patient's feet.

Stabilization: Therapist's trunk and upper extremity stabilize the patient's position.

Mobilization: Patient's head and neck are side bent slightly toward the side to be tested. The patient's head is rotated toward the side to be mobilized so that the T1 segment just begins to move. The lateral side of the therapist's index finger (distal to the metacarpophalangeal joint) is placed over the angle of the first rib with the therapist's forearm positioned in the direction of the movement.

Direction of Force: Therapist produces an anterior, inferior, and medial glide of the first rib.

Cervical-Thoracic Junction (C7/T1–T2/3)

Thoracic Outlet Test: Adson's Test

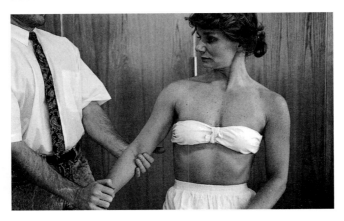

Patient Position: Patient sits.

Therapist Position: Therapist stands facing the patient on the side to be tested.

Stabilization: Provided by the patient's body weight.

Mobilization: Patient is instructed to turn his/her head toward the side to be tested, tuck his/her chin down and in, dorsal glide his/her head back, and to inhale deeply. Therapist monitors the patient's radial pulse at the wrist with the shoulder in a neutral position.

Direction of Force: Cervical rotation and axial extension during inhalation.

Positive findings include a change in the radial pulse (a decrease, absence, change in strength, or disappearance) and provocation of the symptoms.

Cervical-Thoracic Junction (C7/T1–T2/3)

Thoracic Outlet Test: Costoclavicular Test

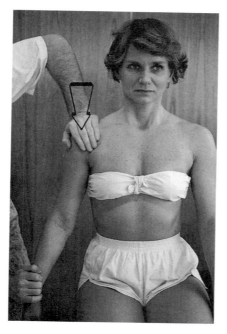

Patient Position: Patient sits.

Therapist Position: Therapist stands facing the patient on the side to be tested.

Stabilization: Provided by the patient's body weight.

Mobilization: Therapist passively depresses the patient's shoulder girdle and asks the patient to inhale. Therapist palpates the radial pulse at the wrist with the shoulder in a neutral position.

Direction of Force: Shoulder girdle depression during inhalation.

Positive findings include a change in the radial pulse (a decrease, absence, change in strength, or disappearance) and provocation of the symptoms.

Cervical-Thoracic Junction (C7/T1–T2/3)

Thoracic Outlet Test: Pectoralis Minor Test

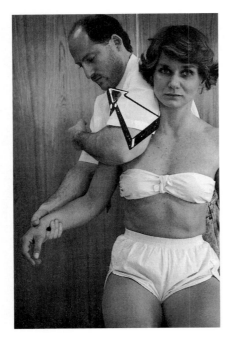

Patient Position: Patient sits.

Therapist Position: Therapist stands behind the patient facing the side to be tested.

Stabilization: Therapist's trunk supports the posterior thorax on the side to be tested.

Mobilization: Therapist palpates the patient's radial pulse at the wrist while passively elevating and retracting the patient's shoulder girdle with the therapist's opposite arm. Patient actively retracts the shoulder girdle at the same time (inhaling) and then exhales completely.

Direction of Force: Shoulder girdle retraction and elevation during exhalation.

Positive findings include a change in the radial pulse (a decrease, absence, change in strength, or disappearance) and provocation of the symptoms.

Cervical (C2/3–C6/7)

Passive Physiologic Segmental Movement Testing: Forward Bending

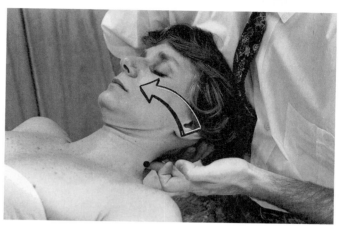

Patient Position: Patient lies supine with the head/neck off the edge of the table in a neutral resting position.

Therapist Position: Therapist stands or sits at the head of the patient.

Stabilization: Provided by the patient's body weight.

Mobilization: Therapist's one hand supports the patient's occiput. The other hand palpates the facet joint on the opposite side at the level assessed.

Direction of Force: Therapist moves the patient's head up and forward through an arc of flexion. This technique should be repeated on both sides to assess the amount of flexion available at motion segments C2/3 through C6/7.

Cervical (C2/3-C6/7)

Passive Physiologic Segmental Movement Testing: Backward Bending

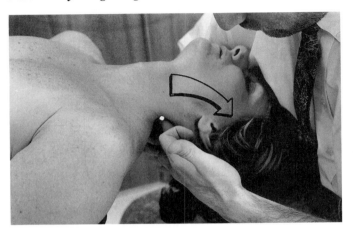

Patient Position: Patient lies supine with the head/neck off the edge of the table in a neutral resting position.

Therapist Position: Therapist stands or sits at the head of the patient.

Stabilization: Provided by the patient's body weight.

Mobilization: Therapist's one hand supports the occiput. The other hand palpates the facet joint on the opposite side at the level assessed.

Direction of Force: Therapist moves the patient's head down and backward through an arc of extension. This technique should be repeated on both sides to assess the amount of extension available at motion segments C2/3 through C6/7.

Cervical (C2/3–C6/7)

Passive Physiologic Segmental Movement Testing: Side Bending

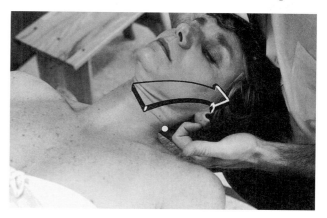

Patient Position: Patient lies supine with the head/neck off the edge of the table in a neutral resting position.

Therapist Position: Therapist stands or sits at the head of the patient.

Stabilization: Provided by the patient's body weight.

Mobilization: Therapist's right hand supports the patient's occiput. The left hand palpates the facet joint on the left side at the level assessed.

Direction of Force: Therapist moves the patient's head to the left through an arc of side bending. This technique should also be repeated to the right side to assess the amount of side bending available at motion segments C2/3 through C6/7.

Cervical (C2/3–C6/7)

Passive Physiologic Segmental Movement Testing: Rotation

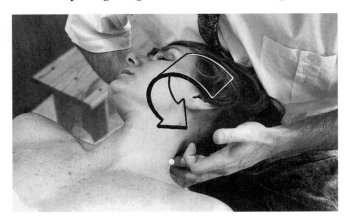

Patient Position: Patient lies supine with the head/neck off the edge of the table in a neutral resting position.

Therapist Position: Therapist stands or sits at the head of the patient.

Stabilization: Provided by the patient's body weight.

Mobilization: Therapist's right hand supports the patient's occiput and the therapist's trunk supports the top of the patient's head. The left hand palpates the facet joint on the left side at the level assessed.

Direction of Force: Therapist moves the patient's head to the right through an arc of rotation. This technique should also be repeated to the left side to assess the amount of rotation available at motion segments C2/3 through C6/7.

Cervical (C2/3–C6/7)

Passive Accessory Movement Testing: Side Gliding

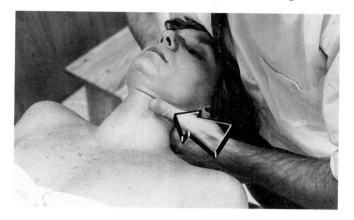

Patient Position: Patient lies supine with the head/neck off the edge of the table in a neutral resting position.

Therapist Position: Therapist stands or sits at the head of the patient.

Stabilization: Provided by the patient's body weight.

Mobilization: Therapist's right hand supports the patient's occiput and the therapist's trunk supports the top of the patient's head. The index finger and web space of the left hand are placed over the articular pillar (posterior arch) of C2 on the left. The left forearm is aligned perpendicular to the cervical spine.

Direction of Force: Therapist applies force through the left hand gliding C2 to the right. The head should remain in neutral and travel with the segment to be moved. Piccolo traction of the neck is given by the right hand. This technique should be repeated C2 through C6 and compared to the left side.

This technique increases diastolic and systolic blood pressure, heart rate, and respiratory rate significantly more (p<0.05) than does a placebo or a control condition.[7]

Cervical (C2/3–C6/7)

Passive Accessory Movement Testing: Central Posterior-Anterior Pressure

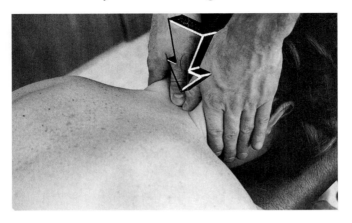

Patient Position: Patient lies prone with the spine in a neutral position.

Therapist Position: Therapist stands at the head of the patient in the midline.

Stabilization: Provided by the patient's body weight and the table.

Mobilization: Therapist places both thumbs over the spinous process of C2 through C6. The other fingers of both hands are placed over the anterolateral aspects of the segment to be moved.

Direction of Force: Therapist pushes down with the thumbs in an anterior direction and then lifts up with the fingers to the starting position. This technique is repeated from C2 through C6.

Cervical (C2/3–C6/7)

Passive Accessory Movement Testing: Unilateral Posterior-Anterior Pressure

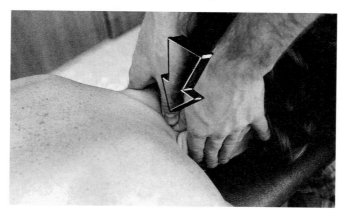

Patient Position: Patient lies prone with the spine in a neutral position.

Therapist Position: Therapist stands at the head of the patient slightly to the left.

Stabilization: Provided by the patient's body weight and the table.

Mobilization: Therapist places both thumbs over the left posterior arch (C2 through C6). The other fingers of both hands are placed over the anterolateral aspect of the segment to be moved.

Direction of Force: Therapist pushes down with both thumbs in an anterior direction and then lifts up with the fingers to the starting position. This technique is repeated on the right side of C2 through C6.

Cervical (C2/3–C6/7)

Specific Quadrant Position Testing (C2-C6)

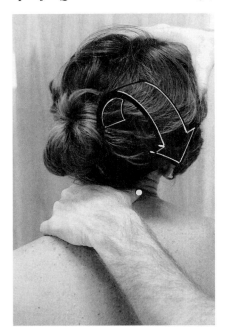

Patient Position: Patient sits with the feet supported.

Therapist Position: Therapist stands behind the patient off to the right side.

Stabilization: Therapist places the left thumb/thenar eminence over the right posterior arch of C3.

Mobilization: Therapist's right hand grasps the top of the patient's head off to the right side.

Direction of Force: Therapist guides the patient's head into right rotation, right side bending, and backward bending simultaneously. This movement takes place down to the C2/3 motion segment. This technique is repeated for each cervical motion segment below C3 (for example: stabilize C4 and move C3, stabilize C5 and move C4, and so on) and to the opposite side.

Cervical (C2/3–C6/7)

Vertebral Artery Testing

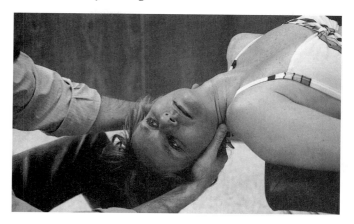

This is a special test for the integrity of the vertebral artery. The following positioning may compromise vertebral artery blood flow.

Patient Position: Patient lies supine with the head/neck off the edge of the table in a neutral resting position.

Therapist Position: Therapist stands or sits at the head of the patient.

Stabilization: Patient's body weight and the table provide stabilization.

Mobilization: Therapist places a hand over the posterolateral aspect of each side of the patient's head.

Direction of Force: Therapist slowly lowers the patient's head into rotation right, side bending right, and backward bending simultaneously. This position should be pain free and is held for approximately 10 seconds.

A positive test may be determined by the provocation of one or more of the following: dizziness (the most common and most predominant symptom; and it might be the only symptom); diplopia; dysarthria; dysphagia; drop attack; nausea; faintness; nystagmus; hemianesthesia; and/or hemiplegia. The test is held until the therapist believes that the test is negative (up to 1 minute).[8]

A negative vertebral artery test may not conclusively indicate adequate profusion by the vertebral arteries, but may reflect normal profusion via collateral circulation.[9]

Upper Cervical (Occiput—C1/2)

Active Movement Testing: Forward Bending Occiput-Atlas

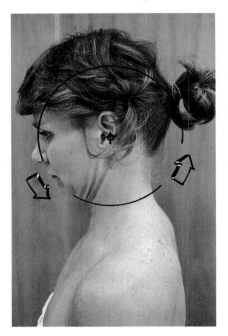

Observe the patient standing or sitting from an anterior, a posterior, and both lateral views. Note any asymmetries using major landmarks and differences in the two positions.

Patient Position: Patient sits with the trunk and the head in a neutral position.

Therapist Position: Therapist stands and observes the patient's motion.

Direction of Force: Patient actively produces forward bending of the occiput on atlas by tucking his/her chin down and in (the axis is through the external auditory meatus in the frontal plane).

Ask questions regarding the reproduction of symptoms while observing the quality and quantity of active movements. Assess the movements from the top down, noting segmental recruitment of motion. Identify deviations from the normal planes of motion including rotation, side bending, forward, or backward bending, flexion, or extension.

Upper Cervical (Occiput—C1/2)

Occiput-Atlas Overpressure: Forward Bending

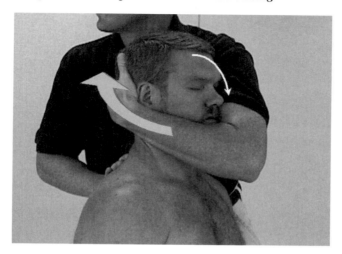

Patient Position: Patient sits with the trunk and the head in a neutral position.

Therapist Position: Therapist stands alongside the patient.

Stabilization: Provided by the patient's body weight and by one of the therapist's hands at the C7 area.

Mobilization: Therapist grasps the occiput around the contralateral side of the patient's head.

Direction of Force: Therapist dorsally glides the patient's head on neck.

Upper Cervical (Occiput—C1/2)

Active Movement Testing: Backward Bending Occiput-Atlas

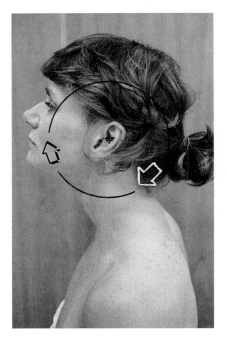

Observe the patient standing or sitting from an anterior, a posterior, and both lateral views. Note any asymmetries using major landmarks and differences in the two positions.

Patient Position: Patient sits with the trunk and the head in a neutral position.

Therapist Position: Therapist stands and observes the patient's motion.

Direction of Force: Patient actively produces backward bending by lifting his/her chin up and forward (the axis is through the external auditory meatus in the frontal plane).

Ask questions regarding the reproduction of symptoms while observing the quality and quantity of active movements. Assess the movements from the top down, noting segmental recruitment of motion. Identify deviations from the normal planes of motion including rotation, side bending, forward, or backward bending.

Upper Cervical (Occiput—C1/2)

Occiput-Atlas Overpressure: Backward Bending

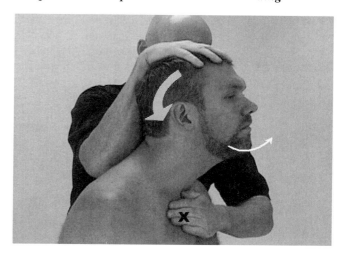

Patient Position: Patient sits with the trunk and the head in a neutral position.

Therapist Position: Therapist stands alongside the patient.

Stabilization: Provided by the patient's body weight and by one of the therapist's hands at the patient's sternum.

Mobilization: Therapist's other hand grasps the vertex of the patient's head with the therapist's forearm resting along the patient's occiput.

Direction of Force: Therapist extends the patient's head on neck.

Upper Cervical (Occiput—C1/2)

Active Movement Testing: Side Bending/Rotation Occiput-Atlas

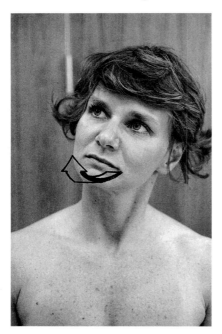

Observe the patient standing or sitting from an anterior, a posterior, and both lateral views. Note any asymmetries using major landmarks and differences in the two positions.

Patient Position: Patient sits with the trunk and the head in a neutral position.

Therapist Position: Therapist stands and observes the patient's motion.

Direction of Force: Patient actively produces side bending with rotation in the opposite direction of the occiput on atlas by side bending the head while lifting the chin to the opposite side in a U-shaped movement (the axis is through the nose in the sagittal plane).

Ask questions regarding the reproduction of symptoms while observing the quality and quantity of active movements. Assess the movements from the top down, noting segmental recruitment of motion. Identify deviations from the normal planes of motion including rotation, side bending, forward, or backward bending.

Upper Cervical (Occiput—C1/2)

Active Movement Testing: Rotation Atlas-Axis; Forward Bend Lock

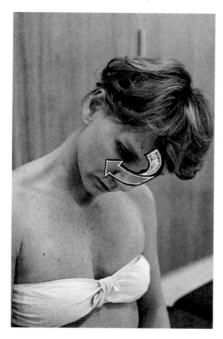

Observe the patient standing or sitting from an anterior, a posterior, and both lateral views. Note any asymmetries using major landmarks and differences in the two positions.

Patient Position: Patient sits with the trunk and the head in a neutral position.

Therapist Position: Therapist stands and observes the patient's motion.

Direction of Force: Patient actively fully flexes his/her cervical spine (ligamentous locking of the mid-cervical spine) and then maximally axially rotates. The range of motion is compared to the opposite side.

Ask questions regarding the reproduction of symptoms while observing the quality and quantity of active movements. Assess the movements from the top down, noting segmental recruitment of motion. Identify deviations from the normal planes of motion including rotation, side bending, forward, or backward bending.

Upper Cervical (Occiput—C1/2)

Active Movement Testing: Rotation Atlas-Axis; Side Bend Lock

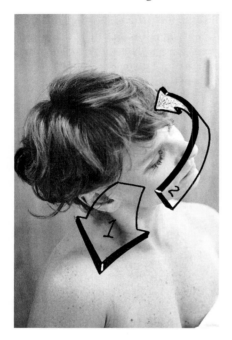

Observe the patient standing or sitting from an anterior, a posterior, and both lateral views. Note any asymmetries using major landmarks and differences in the two positions.

Patient Position: Patient sits with the trunk and the head in a neutral position.

Therapist Position: Therapist stands and observes the patient's motion.

Direction of Force: Patient actively fully side bends his/her cervical spine (facet locking of the mid-cervical spine) and then maximally axially rotates. The range of motion is compared to the opposite side.

Ask questions regarding the reproduction of symptoms while observing the quality and quantity of active movements. Assess the movements from the top down, noting segmental recruitment of motion. Identify deviations from the normal planes of motion including rotation, side bending, forward, or backward bending.

Upper Cervical (Occiput—C1/2)

Passive Movement Testing/Overpressure: Rotation Atlas-Axis; Forward Bend Lock

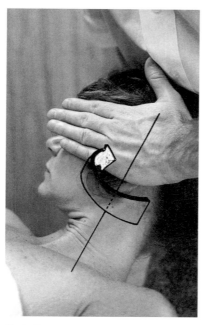

Patient Position: Patient lies supine with the head and the neck positioned over the edge of the table.

Therapist Position: Therapist stands toward the head of the patient resting the patient's head on the therapist's abdomen.

Stabilization: Therapist cradles the patient's occiput with one hand. The palm of the other hand is placed over the temporal region on the side opposite to which rotation will occur.

Mobilization: Therapist passively flexes the cervical spine maximally on the trunk followed by full passive axial rotation. Comparison is made to the opposite side.

Direction of Force: Rotation of the atlas.

Upper Cervical (Occiput—C1/2)

Passive Movement Testing/Overpressure: Rotation Atlas-Axis; Side Bend Lock

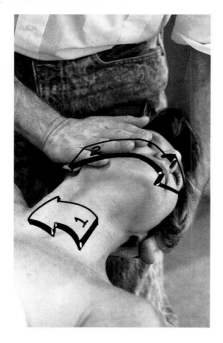

Patient Position: Patient lies supine with the head and the neck over the edge of the table.

Therapist Position: Therapist stands at the head of the table facing the patient.

Stabilization: Provided by the patient's body weight.

Direction of Force: Therapist side bends the cervical spine to end range in one direction. Maintaining side bending, the head is then rotated in the other direction.

Because C1/2 has no appreciable side bending and the other cervical segments do, most of the rotation that takes place should be from the atlas.

Upper Cervical (Occiput—C1/2)

Passive Physiologic Segmental Movement Testing: Forward Bending Occiput-Atlas

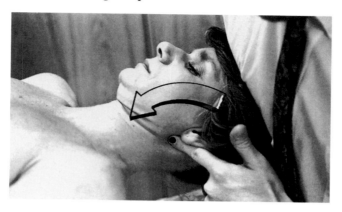

Patient Position: Patient lies supine with the head and the neck positioned over the edge of the table.

Therapist Position: Therapist sits at the head of the patient.

Stabilization: Therapist stabilizes the vertex of the patient's head lightly against the chest or abdomen of the therapist.

Mobilization: Therapist supports the patient's occiput with one hand while palpating the transverse process of the atlas and the mastoid process with a finger of the other hand.

Direction of Force: Therapist passively forward bends the occiput on the atlas, notes the relative increase in distance and soft tissue tension between the atlas and mastoid, and compares the findings to the opposite side.

Upper Cervical (Occiput—C1/2)

Passive Physiologic Segmental Movement Testing: Backward Bending Occiput-Atlas

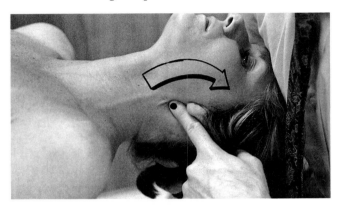

Patient Position: Patient lies supine with the head and the neck positioned over the edge of the table.

Therapist Position: Therapist sits at the head of the patient.

Stabilization: Therapist stabilizes the vertex of the patient's head lightly against the chest or abdomen of the therapist.

Mobilization: Therapist supports the patient's occiput with one hand while palpating the transverse process of the atlas and the mastoid process with a finger of the other hand.

Direction of Force: Therapist passively backward bends the occiput on the atlas, notes the relative decrease in distance and soft tissue relaxation between the atlas and mastoid, and compares the findings to the opposite side.

Upper Cervical (Occiput—C1/2)

Passive Physiologic Segmental Movement Testing:
Side Bending Occiput-Atlas

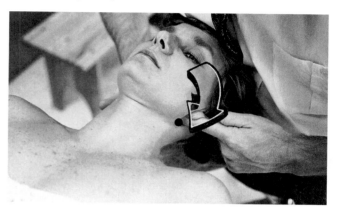

Patient Position: Patient lies supine with the head and the neck positioned over the edge of the table.

Therapist Position: Therapist sits at the head of the patient.

Stabilization: Therapist stabilizes the vertex of the patient's head lightly against the chest or abdomen of the therapist.

Mobilization: Therapist supports the patient's occiput with one hand while palpating the transverse process of the atlas and the mastoid process with a finger of the other hand to which the side bending occurs.

Direction of Force: Therapist passively side bends the occiput on the atlas, notes the transverse process of the atlas move into the palpating finger, and compares the findings to the opposite side.

Upper Cervical (Occiput—C1/2)

Passive Physiologic Segmental Movement Testing: Rotation Occiput-Atlas

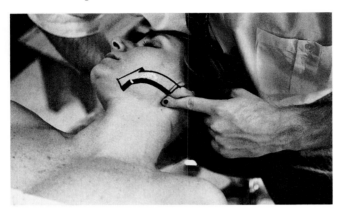

Patient Position: Patient lies supine with the head and the neck positioned over the edge of the table.

Therapist Position: Therapist sits at the head of the patient.

Stabilization: Therapist stabilizes the vertex of the patient's head lightly against the chest or abdomen of the therapist.

Mobilization: Therapist supports the patient's occiput with one hand while palpating the transverse process of the atlas and the mastoid process with a finger of the other hand.

Direction of Force: Therapist passively rotates the occiput on the atlas away from the palpating finger, notes the relative increase in distance and soft tissue tension between the atlas and mastoid, and compares the findings to the opposite side.

Upper Cervical (Occiput—C1/2)

*Passive Physiologic Segmental Movement Testing:
Forward Bending Atlas-Axis*

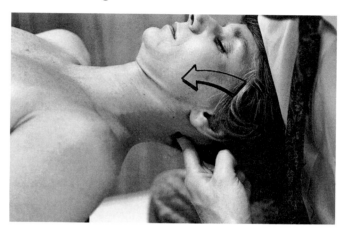

Patient Position: Patient lies supine with the head and the neck positioned over the edge of the table.

Therapist Position: Therapist sits at the head of the patient.

Stabilization: Therapist stabilizes the vertex of the patient's head lightly against the chest or abdomen of the therapist.

Mobilization: Therapist supports the patient's occiput with one hand while palpating the posterior arch of C1 with a finger of the other hand.

Direction of Force: Therapist passively forward bends the atlas on the axis, notes the relative anterior motion of the C1 lamina and the corresponding increase in soft tissue tension, and compares the findings to the opposite side.

Upper Cervical (Occiput—C1/2)

Passive Physiologic Segmental Movement Testing:
Backward Bending Atlas-Axis

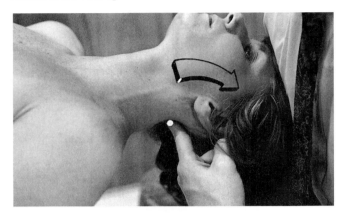

Patient Position: Patient lies supine with the head and the neck positioned over the edge of the table.

Therapist Position: Therapist sits at the head of the patient.

Stabilization: Therapist stabilizes the vertex of the patient's head lightly against the chest or abdomen of the therapist.

Mobilization: Therapist supports the patient's occiput with one hand while palpating the posterior arch of C1 with a finger of the other hand.

Direction of Force: Therapist passively backward bends the atlas on the axis, notes the relative posterior motion of the C1 lamina and the corresponding soft tissue relaxation, and compares the findings to the opposite side.

Upper Cervical (Occiput—C1/2)

Passive Physiologic Segmental Movement Testing: Rotation Atlas-Axis

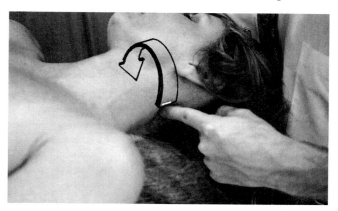

Patient Position: Patient lies supine with the head and the neck positioned over the edge of the table.

Therapist Position: Therapist sits at the head of the patient.

Stabilization: Therapist stabilizes the vertex of the patient's head lightly against the chest or abdomen of the therapist.

Mobilization: Therapist supports the patient's occiput with one hand while palpating the posterior arch of C1 with a finger of the other hand.

Direction of Force: Therapist passively rotates the atlas on the axis away from the palpating finger, notes the relative anterior motion of C1 and the corresponding increase in soft tissue tension, and compares the findings to the opposite side.

Upper Cervical (Occiput—C1/2)

Passive Accessory Movement Testing: Central Posterior-Anterior Pressure; Atlas

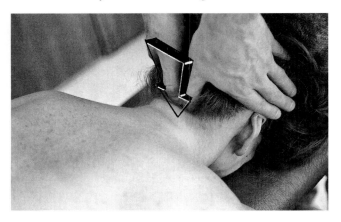

Patient Position: Patient lies prone in a neutral cervical position.

Therapist Position: Therapist stands at the head of the patient.

Stabilization: Provided by the table.

Mobilization: Therapist places both thumb tips over the posterior tubercle of the atlas with the thumb pads facing cephalically.

Direction of Force: Therapist produces an anteriorly directed force on the atlas.

Indications: Positive pain reproduction with upper motor neuron lesion signs—such as extrasegmental pins and needles; 3+/4+ reflexes with clonus; positive cutaneous reflex(es); ataxic-like gait; bowel or bladder incontinence; or perineum sensory changes—may indicate a dens fracture or transverse ligament rupture.

Upper Cervical (Occiput—C1/2)

Passive Accessory Movement Testing: Central Posterior-Anterior Pressure; Axis

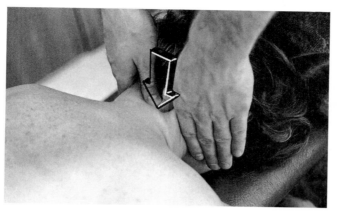

Patient Position: Patient lies prone in a neutral cervical position.

Therapist Position: Therapist stands at the head of the patient.

Stabilization: Provided by the table.

Mobilization: Therapist places both thumb tips over the spinous process of C2. The other fingers of both hands are placed over the anterolateral aspects of the segment to be moved.

Direction of Force: Therapist produces an anteriorly directed force on the axis.

Indications: Positive pain reproduction with upper motor neuron lesion signs—such as extrasegmental pins and needles; 3+/4+ reflexes with clonus; positive cutaneous reflex(es); ataxic-like gait; bowel or bladder incontinence; or perineum sensory changes—may indicate a fracture of the anterior arch of C1 or a dens fracture.

Upper Cervical (Occiput—C1/2)

Passive Accessory Movement Testing: Unilateral Posterior-Anterior Pressure; Atlas

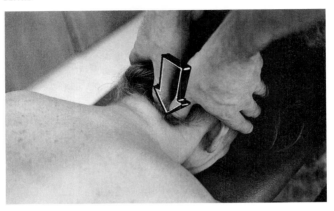

Patient Position: Patient lies prone in a neutral cervical position.

Therapist Position: Therapist stands at the head of the patient.

Stabilization: Provided by the table.

Mobilization: Therapist places both thumb tips on the posterior arch of the atlas with the thumb pads facing cephalically.

Direction of Force: Therapist produces an anteriorly directed force and compares this motion to the opposite side.

Upper Cervical (Occiput—C1/2)

Passive Accessory Movement Testing: Unilateral Posterior-Anterior Pressure; Axis

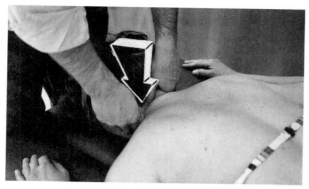

Patient Position: Patient lies prone in a neutral cervical position.

Therapist Position: Therapist stands at the head of the patient.

Stabilization: Provided by the table.

Mobilization: Both thumbs are placed on one side of the posterior arch of the axis with thumb pads facing away from each other.

Direction of Force: Therapist produces an anteriorly directed force and compares this motion to the opposite side.

Patient's head can be rotated approximately 30° toward one side. A similar posterior-anterior pressure can be exerted on the right side of the posterior arch (figure below) to specifically increase the rotation occurring between the atlas and the axis.

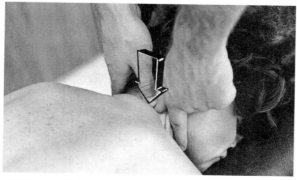

Unilateral Axis Posterior-Anterior Pressure with Rotation

Upper Cervical (Occiput—C1/2)

Passive Accessory Movement Testing: Transverse Vertebral Pressure; Atlas

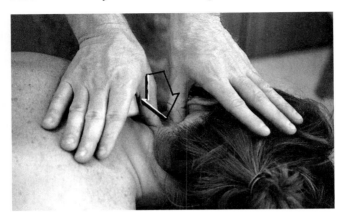

Patient Position: Patient lies prone with the head rotated approximately 30°.

Therapist Position: Therapist stands at the side toward which rotation has occurred.

Stabilization: Provided by the table.

Mobilization: The tips of both thumbs are placed onto the lateral tip of the transverse process of C1 with the thumb pads facing away from each other.

Direction of Force: Therapist produces a transversely directed force on the atlas moving down toward the table in a line parallel with the suboccipital line.

Indication: A left transverse pressure (figure above) for a right side bending hypomobility.

Upper Cervical (Occiput—C1/2)

Alar Ligament Test

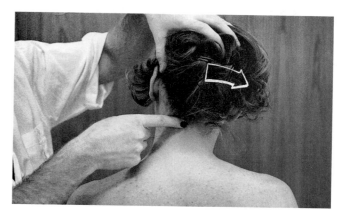

This is a special test for the stability of the occiput-atlas-axis complex.

Patient Position: Patient sits.

Therapist Position: Therapist faces the patient on his/her lateral side.

Stabilization: Therapist places one hand on the vertex of the cranium.

Mobilization: Therapist palpates immediately lateral to the C2 spinous process (ipsilateral side, left in the figure) while controlling side bending of the occiput.

Direction of Force: Therapist side bends the cranium on the spine away from the side of palpation (right in the figure).

Indication: Side bending of the cranium normally should produce immediate rotation of the C2 spinous process in the opposite direction. Lack of immediate rotation following cranial side bending is suggestive of alar ligament laxity.

Temporomandibular Joint (TMJ)

Active Movement Testing/Overpressure: Opening

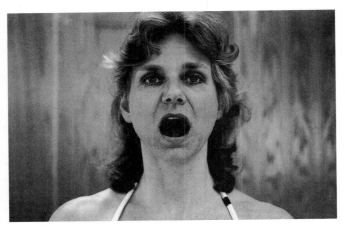

Observe the patient standing or sitting from an anterior, a posterior, and both lateral views. Note any asymmetries using major landmarks and differences in the two positions.

Patient Position: Patient stands or sits in a neutral posture for active movements and lies supine for an overpressure.

Therapist Position: Therapist stands and observes the patient's active movement. During active movements the therapist can palpate the temporomandibular joint laterally (top figure page 361) or the posterior capsule within the external auditory meatus (EAM) (middle figure page 361). The therapist sits/stands at the patient's head during the overpressure.

Stabilization: One of the therapist's hands cradles the patient's neck during the overpressure.

Mobilization: The therapist's other hand grasps the mandible at the jaw during the overpressure.

Direction of Force: Therapist passively opens the patient's temporomandibular joint (bottom figure page 361).

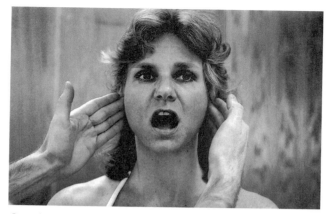

Opening Active Movement TMJ Palpation

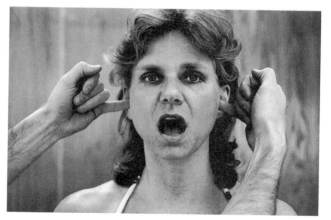

Opening Active Movement EAM Palpation

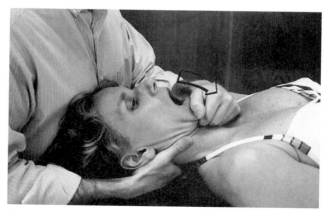

Opening Overpressure

Temporomandibular Joint (TMJ)

Active Movement Testing: Closing/Retrusion

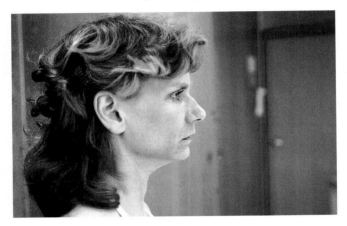

Observe the patient standing or sitting from an anterior, a posterior, and both lateral views. Note any asymmetries using major landmarks and differences in the two positions.

Patient Position: Patient stands or sits in a neutral posture for active movements.

Therapist Position: Therapist stands and observes the patient's active movement.

Stabilization: Provided by the patient's body weight.

Direction of Force: Patient actively retrudes the temporomandibular joint to the end of range.

Temporomandibular Joint (TMJ)

Active Movement Testing/Overpressure: Protrusion

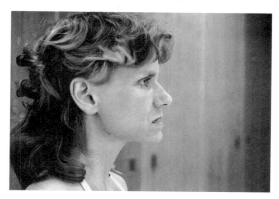

Observe the patient standing or sitting from an anterior, a posterior, and both lateral views. Note any asymmetries using major landmarks and differences in the two positions.

Patient Position: Patient stands or sits in a neutral posture for active movements and lies supine for an overpressure.

Therapist Position: Therapist stands and observes the patient's active movement. The therapist sits/stands at the patient's head during the overpressure.

Stabilization: Provided by the patient's body weight.

Mobilization: Both of the therapist's hands grasp the angle of the mandible on either side of the patient's head during the overpressure.

Direction of Force: Therapist passively protrudes the temporomandibular joint.

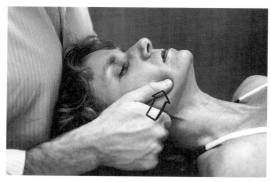

Protrusion Overpressure

Temporomandibular Joint (TMJ)

Active Movement Testing/Overpressure: Lateral Glide

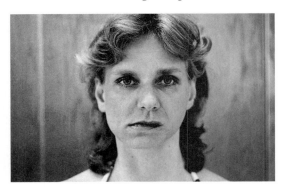

Observe the patient standing or sitting from an anterior, a posterior, and both lateral views. Note any asymmetries using major landmarks and differences in the two positions.

Patient Position: Patient stands or sits in a neutral posture for active movements and lies supine for an overpressure.

Therapist Position: Therapist stands and observes the patient's active movement. The therapist sits/stands at the patient's head during the overpressure.

Stabilization: One of the therapist's hands cradles the patient's head and the lateral side of the face during the overpressure.

Mobilization: The other therapist's hand grasps the mandible opposite to the stabilization hand during the overpressure.

Direction of Force: Therapist passively glides the mandible laterally.

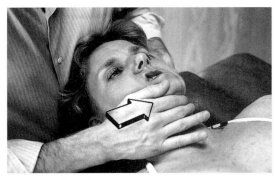

Lateral Glide Overpressure

Temporomandibular Joint (TMJ)

Passive Accessory Movement Testing: Distraction (Nonweight Bearing)

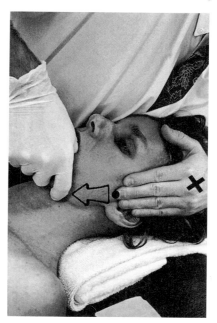

Patient Position: Patient lies supine with the neck supported in a neutral position.

Therapist Position: Therapist stands to the side of the patient's head opposite to the TMJ to be tested.

Stabilization: Therapist's trunk and the cephalic hand support the patient's head while palpating the TMJ.

Mobilization: Therapist's caudal thumb is placed intraorally on top of the bottom row of teeth on the side of the TMJ to be assessed as far back as possible. Therapist's fingers and hand support the outside of the mandible.

Direction of Force: Therapist's caudal arm and hand move in a caudal direction with the force coming through the thumb over the lower teeth.

Indication: Any capsular hypomobility.

Temporomandibular Joint (TMJ)

Passive Accessory Movement Testing: Compression (Nonweight Bearing)

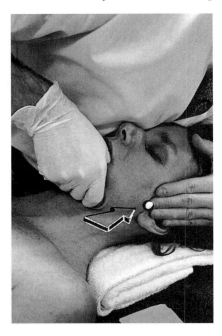

Patient Position: Patient lies supine with the neck supported in a neutral position.

Therapist Position: Therapist stands to the side of the patient's head opposite to the TMJ to be tested.

Stabilization: Therapist's trunk and cephalic hand support the patient's head while palpating the TMJ.

Mobilization: Therapist's caudal thumb is placed intraorally on top of the bottom row of teeth on the side of the TMJ to be assessed as far back as possible. Therapist's fingers and hand support the outside of the mandible.

Direction of Force: Therapist's caudal arm and hand move in a cephalic direction with the force coming through the hand on the mandible.

Indication: Provocation finding with arthritis.[1]

Temporomandibular Joint (TMJ)

Passive Accessory Movement Testing: Anterior Glide (Nonweight Bearing)

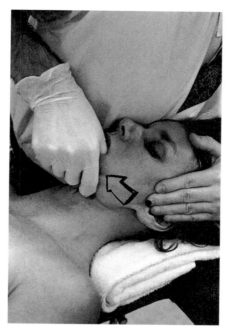

Patient Position: Patient lies supine with the neck supported in a neutral position.

Therapist Position: Therapist stands to the side of the patient's head opposite to the TMJ to be tested.

Stabilization: Therapist's trunk and cephalic hand support the patient's head while palpating the TMJ.

Mobilization: Therapist's caudal thumb is placed intraorally over the bottom row of teeth on the side of the TMJ to be assessed as far back as possible. Therapist's fingers and hand grasp around the bottom of the mandible.

Direction of Force: Therapist's caudal arm and hand pull the mandible forward (anteriorly) and medially.

Indications: Protrusion hypomobility and opening hypomobility.

Temporomandibular Joint (TMJ)

Passive Accessory Movement Testing: Posterior Glide (Nonweight Bearing)

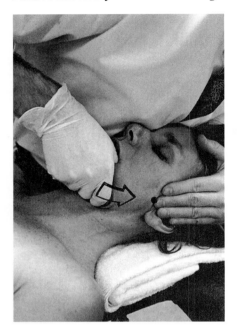

Patient Position: Patient lies supine with the neck supported in a neutral position.

Therapist Position: Therapist stands to the side of the patient's head opposite to the TMJ to be tested.

Stabilization: Therapist's trunk and cephalic hand support the patient's head while palpating the TMJ.

Mobilization: Therapist's caudal thumb is placed intraorally over the bottom row of teeth on the side of the TMJ to be assessed as far back as possible. Therapist's fingers and hand grasp around the bottom of the mandible.

Direction of Force: Therapist's caudal arm and hand push the mandible backward (posteriorly) and laterally.

Indication: Retrusion hypomobility.

Temporomandibular Joint (TMJ)

Passive Accessory Movement Testing: Medial Glide (Nonweight Bearing)

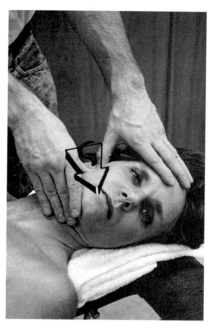

Patient Position: Patient lies supine with the neck supported and the head rotated away from the therapist and supported.

Therapist Position: Therapist stands on the same side of the patient's head as the TMJ to be tested.

Stabilization: Fingers of the therapist's cephalic hand on the patient's forehead and a towel roll under the patient's head provide stabilization.

Mobilization: Therapist places both thumbs over the ramus of the mandible near the joint line. Therapist's fingers of the caudal hand gently support the mandible in a neutral position.

Direction of Force: Therapist applies force in a medial direction with the thumbs.

Indication: Medial glide hypomobility.

Temporomandibular Joint (TMJ)

Passive Accessory Movement Testing: Lateral Glide (Nonweight Bearing)

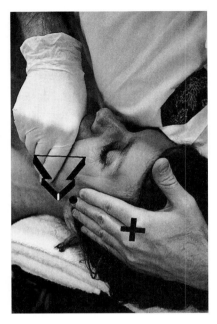

Patient Position: Patient lies supine with the neck supported in a neutral position.

Therapist Position: Therapist stands to the side of the patient's head opposite to the TMJ to be tested.

Stabilization: Therapist's trunk and cephalic hand support the patient's head while palpating the TMJ.

Mobilization: Therapist's caudal thumb is placed in the patient's mouth along the medial border of the mandible. It should be below the teeth with the pad of the thumb over the ramus of the mandible. Therapist's fingers and hand grasp around the outside of the mandible laterally.

Direction of Force: Therapist's caudal arm and hand push the mandible laterally with the force coming through the thumb.

Indication: Lateral glide hypomobility.

A medial glide can also be done by pulling the mandible toward the therapist with the fingers (not pictured).

Indication: Medial glide hypomobility.

Temporomandibular Joint (TMJ)

Passive Accessory Movement Testing: Distraction (Weight Bearing)

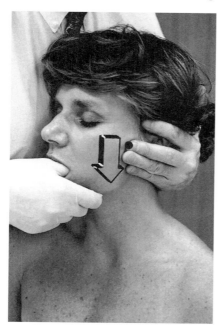

Patient Position: Patient sits with the head/neck in a neutral position.

Therapist Position: Therapist stands to the side of the patient's head opposite to the TMJ to be tested.

Stabilization: Therapist's trunk and posterior hand support the patient's head while palpating the TMJ.

Mobilization: Therapist places the thumb of the anterior hand intraorally over the bottom row of teeth on the side of the TMJ to be assessed as far back as possible. Therapist's fingers and hand grasp around the bottom of the mandible.

Direction of Force: Therapist's anterior arm and hand pull the mandible down in a caudal direction with the force coming through the thumb.

Indication: Any capsular hypomobility.

Temporomandibular Joint (TMJ)

Passive Accessory Movement Testing: Compression (Weight Bearing)

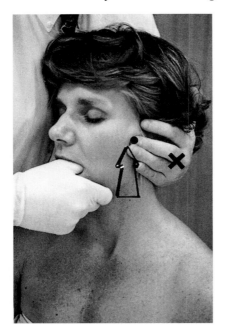

Patient Position: Patient sits with the head/neck in a neutral position.

Therapist Position: Therapist stands to the side of the patient's head opposite to the TMJ to be tested.

Stabilization: Therapist's trunk and posterior hand support the patient's head while palpating the TMJ.

Mobilization: Therapist places the thumb of the anterior hand intraorally over the bottom row of teeth on the side of the TMJ to be assessed as far back as possible. Therapist's fingers and hand grasp around the bottom of the mandible.

Direction of Force: Therapist's anterior arm and hand lift the mandible up in a cephalic direction with the force coming through the fingers.

Indication: Provocation findings with arthritis.[1]

Temporomandibular Joint (TMJ)

Passive Accessory Movement Testing: Anterior Glide (Weight Bearing)

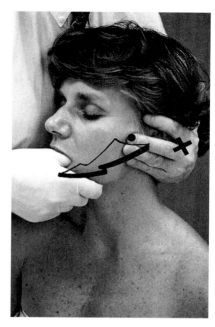

Patient Position: Patient sits with the head/neck in a neutral position.

Therapist Position: Therapist stands to the side of the patient's head opposite to the TMJ to be tested.

Stabilization: Therapist's trunk and posterior hand support the patient's head while palpating the TMJ.

Mobilization: Therapist places the thumb of the anterior hand intraorally over the bottom row of teeth on the side of the TMJ to be assessed as far back as possible. Therapist's fingers and hand grasp around the bottom of the mandible.

Direction of Force: Therapist's anterior arm and hand pull the mandible forward (anteriorly) and medially.

Indications: Protrusion hypomobility and opening hypomobility.

Temporomandibular Joint (TMJ)

Passive Accessory Movement Testing: Posterior Glide (Weight Bearing)

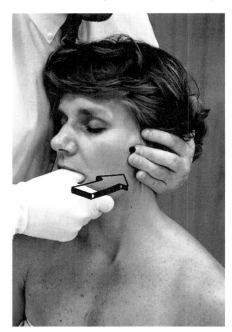

Patient Position: Patient sits with the head/neck in a neutral position.

Therapist Position: Therapist stands to the side of the patient's head opposite to the TMJ to be tested.

Stabilization: Therapist's trunk and posterior hand support the patient's head while palpating the TMJ.

Mobilization: Therapist places the thumb of the anterior hand intraorally over the bottom row of teeth on the side of the TMJ to be assessed as far back as possible. Therapist's fingers and hand grasp around the bottom of the mandible.

Direction of Force: Therapist's anterior arm and hand push the mandible backward (posteriorly) and laterally.

Indication: Retrusion hypomobility.

Temporomandibular Joint (TMJ)

Passive Accessory Movement Testing: Lateral Glide (Weight Bearing)

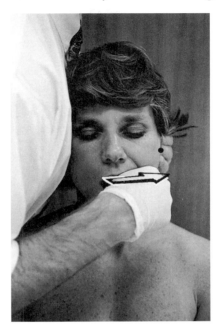

Patient Position: Patient sits with the head/neck in a neutral position.

Therapist Position: Therapist stands to the side of the patient's head opposite to the TMJ to be tested.

Stabilization: Therapist's trunk and posterior hand support the patient's head while palpating the TMJ.

Mobilization: Therapist places the thumb of the anterior hand in the patient's mouth along the medial border of the mandible. It should be below the teeth with the pad of the thumb over the ramus of the mandible. Therapist's fingers and hand grasp around the outside of the mandible laterally.

Direction of Force: Therapist's anterior arm and hand push the mandible laterally with the force coming through the thumb.

Indication: Lateral glide hypomobility.

A medial glide can also be done by pulling the mandible toward the therapist with the fingers (not pictured).

Indication: Medial glide hypomobility.

REFERENCES

1. Cyriax J: Textbook of Orthopaedic Medicine, 8th ed. London, Baillière Tindall, 1982.
2. Magee DJ: Orthopedic Assessment, 3rd ed. Philadelphia, WB Saunders, 1997.
3. Draper DO, Schulthies SS: Examiner proficiency in performing the anterior drawer and Lachman tests. Journal of Orthopaedic & Sports Physical Therapy 22(60):263–266, 1995.
4. Stratford PW, Binkley J: A review of the McMurray test: Definition, interpretation, and clinical usefulness. Journal of Orthopaedic & Sports Physical Therapy 22(3):116–120, 1995.
5. Erhard RE, Bowling RW: The recognition and management of the pelvic component of low back and sciatic pain. Bulletin of the Orthopaedic Section, American Physical Therapy Association 2(3):4–15, 1977.
6. Mitchell FL, Moran PS, Pruzzo NA: An Evaluation and Treatment Manual of Osteopathic Muscle Energy Techniques. Valley Park, MO, Mitchell, Moran, and Pruzzo Associates, 1979.
7. Vicenzino B, Cartwright T, Collins D, Wright: Cardiovascular and respiratory changes produced by lateral glide mobilization of the cervical spine. Manual Therapy 3(2):67–71, 1998.
8. DiFabio RP: Manipulation of the cervical spine: Risks and benefits. Physical Therapy 79(1):50–65, 1999.
9. Rivett DA, Milburn PD, Chapple C: Negative pre-manipulative vertebral artery testing despite complete occlusion: A case of false negativity? Manual Therapy 3(2):102–107, 1998.

PRINCIPLES OF MOBILIZATION FOR INTERVENTION

This chapter discusses the principles of mobilization for intervention using physiologic and accessory motion testing.

APPROACHES TO MOTION RESTRICTION

Three types of techniques — direct, exaggeration, indirect, or a combination of the three — can be used to treat joint movement dysfunction (hypomobility or hypermobility).

The direct technique involves movement into the direction of dysfunction; for example, with a loss of elbow flexion, active or passive movement into elbow flexion is used.

Movement into the opposite direction of the dysfunction is used with the exaggeration method; for example, with a loss of elbow flexion, active or passive movement into elbow extension is the intervention.

Intervention into the least restricted or least painful position is used with the indirect method. This method may work well with hypermobility pain when hypomobility is also present. Typically, areas of hypomobility are found in conjunction with hypermobility. For example, with a hypermobile L5/S1 segment, a hypomobile area may be found in the upper lumbar or thoracic region. By increasing the mobility in the hypomobile area, the hypermobility pain may resolve.

A combination of any of the three techniques can be used. For example, with an acute hypomobile knee extension problem, treatment into knee flexion could be done first (an exaggeration method), followed by movements into knee extension (a direct method).[1 p 96]

CONSIDERATIONS THAT MAY INFLUENCE INTERVENTION

These considerations are not all inclusive but an understanding of how they may affect intervention is important.

Acuity

A general guide is to alleviate inflammation with any acute problem to prevent futher dysfunction. Because swelling is associated with inflammation, the involved tissue may become hypermobile if inflammation is prolonged. Chronic hypomobility problems require techniques that will stretch the hypomobile tissue. Stretching generally aggravates an acute inflammatory problem.

Age

The age of the patient can affect treatment. The growth cartilage in a young child is particularly vulnerable to linear and torsional shears (see Chapter 1, "Indications and Contraindications for Joint Mobilization"). Only gentle oscillations without pain that avoid the ends of range are recommended.[2] Osteoporosis, at any age, must be considered to protect against fracture with any type of end of range technique (movement grades III to V)[3] or stretching.

Patient Condition

The general condition of the patient, including such problems as osteoporosis, diabetes, rheumatoid arthritis, high blood pressure, cardiac disease, menses and pregnancy in females, or general debilitation, can impact intervention; for example, menses or pregnancy in females may put the patient at risk for hypermobility with techniques that move into the end of range due to hormonal laxity.

Pathology

The type of patient pathology may influence the examination; for example, with a spastic hemiparesis patient with shoulder limitations, it may be difficult to differentiate whether the shoulder limitation is capsular in nature or related to the patient's spasticity. With many childhood diagnoses, such as ataxic or spastic cerebral palsy, developmental delay, myelomeningocele, and Down syndrome, cervical instability may be associated.

Patient Interview Information

Information about previous and present treatment including medications, surgeries, and physical therapy may affect intervention choices; for example, if the patient is using steroids, end-range techniques or stretching may cause hypermobility.

Therapist

The therapist's size, strength, or knowledge base may influence intervention; for example, a small therapist may not be able to perform all interventions with a large patient.

Clinical Setting and Equipment

The clinical setting and the equipment available to the therapist enable or limit intervention; for example, from a home healthcare perspective for strengthening activities, equipment availability is limited to what is found in the home (eg, canned goods) or to what can be transported there (eg, weights/sandbags).

TYPES OF ACTIVATING FORCES

What follows are some suggestions for types of forces that can be used to assist intervention.

Active/Active Assistive Range of Motion

Active or active assistive range of motion performed by the patient is generally a safe way to intervene. For instance, to increase thoracic extension, the patient can lean back over a chair.

Respiration

The patient's respiration phases can facilitate motion. Inhalation tends to increase extension in the spine as well as external rotation in the extremities, while exhalation tends to increase flexion in the spine and internal rotation in the extremities.

Muscle Energy

The patient's own muscular force can be used to lengthen a shortened muscle by (a) producing a maximal contraction of the tight muscle to cause maximal relaxation of the tight muscle through autogenic inhibition[4-6] or (b) contraction against resistance through the ends of range using the antagonist to the tight muscle, produces reciprocal inhibition of the tight muscle.[4;7;8]

Passive Motion

Passive techniques performed by the therapist or with equipment (a continuous passive motion machine) can provide physiologic or accessory movement without muscular activation by the patient.

Gravity

Gravity can assist movements; for example, a supine Thomas hip flexor stretch can be performed as a home program.[9]

Inherent Body Forces

The use of inherent subtle body forces, such as the venous system to decrease edema, or cerebrospinal fluid movement with craniosacral therapy, may be altered to affect patients mentally and physically.[10]

INTERVENTION USING GRADES I–V

Maitland's movement grades I to V[3] are a conceptual model for examination of accessory motion and intervention using both physiologic and accessory motions. Additional plus and minus notations can be added to movement grades I to IV; for example, II– and II+ indicate decreased or additional movement respectively, related to the movement grade II technique.

Reference to Figure 1–6 on page 5 is recommended for the information below. For physiologic motion, the beginning range refers to the zero position used to measure goniometric range of motion.[11] Treatment effects can be mechanical or neurologic for each grade of movement.

A grade I movement is a small amplitude movement performed at the beginning of the range of motion. The neurologic treatment effects are greater than the mechanical treatment effects with a grade I movement. The neurologic effects include neuromodulation via the type Ia and II articular receptors.[12 p 948;13] Mechanical effects include minimal joint lubrication, minimal congruency of the joint surfaces, and minimal stress to the joint capsule and ligaments.[14]

A grade II movement is a large amplitude movement performed within the range of motion but not reaching either end of the range of motion. The neurologic treatment effects are greater than the mechanical treatment effects with a grade II movement. The neurologic effects include neuromodulation via the type Ia and II articular receptors. Mechanical effects include increased joint lubrication, an increased area of congruency of articular surfaces, and moderate stress to the joint capsule and ligaments.

Movement grades I and II are free of resistance (stiffness and muscle spasm), so pain should not be reproduced and there is no end-feel to the movement.[3]

A grade III movement is a large amplitude movement that stays off the beginning of the range but that is performed up to the end of the range of motion. The mechanical treatment effects are greater than the neurologic treatment effects with a grade III movement. The mechanical effects include a stretch of the joint capsule and ligaments, increased joint lubrication, and an increased area of congruency of articular surfaces. Neurologic treatment effects include neuromodulation via the types Ia, II, and IIb articular receptors.[12 p 948;13]

A grade IV movement is a small amplitude movement performed at the end of the range of motion. The mechanical treatment effects are greater than the neurologic treatment effects with a grade IV movement. The mechanical effects include a stretch of the joint capsule and ligaments, minimal joint lubrication, and minimal congruency of the joint surfaces. Neurologic treatment effects include neuromodulation via the types Ia, II, and IIb articular receptors.

Movement grades III and IV move into resistance (stiffness and stretch pain) and there is an end-feel to the movement.[3]

A grade V movement is a high velocity, short amplitude thrust (manipulation) performed at the end of the joint play range. The mechanical treatment effects are greater than the neurologic treatment effects with a grade V movement. The mechanical treatment effects include the stretch of soft tissues, tearing of adhesions, and pressure changes in the joint.[15;16] Neurologic treatment effects include neuromodulation via the types Ia, II, and IIb, and possibly III and IV articular receptors.[12 p 948;13]

PRINCIPLES OF INTERVENTION USING PHYSIOLOGIC MOTION

Maitland's movement grades I to IV can be used for intervention[3] (see the specific hypomobility and hypermobility sections in this chapter).

Use the end-feel information in addition to the sequence of pain and resistance (end-feel) to guide intervention. When pathologic end-feels are present, suspect dysfunction.[17] The temporal aspect of examining pain with resistance to determine whether the problem is acute, subacute, or chronic may cause part of the poor reliability found with the pain resistance sequence.[18;19] A spasm end-feel suggests that the joint is not suitable for stretching, but movement grades I and II can be used to neuromodulate the pain.[13] When capsular or early capsular end-feels are found with hypomobility, stretching is the intervention of choice.

PRINCIPLES OF INTERVENTION USING ACCESSORY MOTION

Maitland's movement grades I to V can be used for intervention[3] (see the specific hypomobility and hypermobility sections in this chapter).

Physiologic and accessory motion may be correlated in the extremities based on the concave/convex guidelines and the most normal anatomy in the joint. Recent research (see Chapter 1, Physiologic and Accessory Motion Correlation, page 10) does not support the concave/convex physiologic/accessory motion relationship. Accessory motion interventions should be related to the examination findings and may not be specific to the concave/convex guidelines.

Regarding the specific accessory techniques, distraction is the best technique to stretch the entire joint capsule as when a capsular pattern of limitation is present (see Appendix 4 for a list of capsular patterns for each joint).

Compression is most often used to indicate joint surface changes occuring with arthritides and may be painful when performed. Compression can be used with caution to treat capsular irregularities that may occur with osteoarthritis.[20] The irregularities (an excrescence or a defect) may be smoothed with compression force.

Traction can be used to increase the joint space; for example, to provide relief at the acromioclavicular joint when impingement is present or to decrease weight bearing in the superior portion of the hip joint capsule.

A glide is used to stretch various parts of the capsule determined by (a) the concave convex guidelines (see Chapter 1) or (b) to address any accessory motion limitation found with examination.

Rotation is used to treat any rotational accessory motion problem. All physiologic motion has concomitant conjunct rotation due to the joint's contact areas, tightening of ligaments and muscle contractions.[21;22]

PRINCIPLES OF INTERVENTION FOR HYPOMOBILITY

Using either physiologic or accessory motion, hypomobility due to inflammation or to the subsequent repair process (fibrosis) can be treated with movement grades I to IV (physiologic) or I to V (accessory).

General principles include using movement grades I and II to treat inflammatory problems, and movement grades III to V to treat the fibrosis following repair. Movement grades I and II may be applied subsequent to intervention with the movement grades III to V to resolve treatment discomfort. When pathologic end-feels are present during physiologic motion, there is evidence to suggest pathology is present.[17] A spasm end-feel with physiologic or accessory range of motion suggests an inflammatory process and further motion should not be continued.

There is no evidence to validate that intervention should begin with either physiologic or accessory motion when hypomobility involves both of these types of motion restriction. Normal accessory motion may be necessary to allow normal pain-free physiologic function.[21;23] Clinicians may therefore begin intervention with accessory movements.

Because physiologic motion has a larger excursion of motion compared to accessory motion, physiologic motion may improve the roll that occurs with osteokinematic/arthrokinematic movement.

When using loose- and close-packed positions with accessory motion intervention, it may be best to start in the loose-packed position because the greatest amount of joint play is possible. When no further increase in motion is found in the loose-packed position, progress into the close-packed or restricted physiologic position. There is no evidence for these comments, but biomechanically, the joint is the most mobile in the loose-packed position and the least mobile in the close-packed position.

Guidelines regarding the duration of treatment using the movement grades I to IV include 30- to 90-second bouts, usually continuously performed in 2 to 4 intervention bouts. Reassessment of intervention should occur every 1 to 2 bouts.[3]

Three reassessment decision-making scenarios are: (a) technique A is performed with no change on reassessment; technique A is repeated and again there is no change on reassessment; progress to technique B; (b) technique A is performed with improvement noted on reassessment; continue to use technique A; and (c) technique A is performed with worsening with reassessment; technique A is not repeated, but could be tried later with a change in the patient's symptoms.

In addition to intervention using joint mobilization, any soft tissue technique may be appropriate, such as stretching, deep friction massage, classical massage, and myofascial. Strengthening, posture, ergonomics, and functional movement may need to be addressed as well.

PRINCIPLES OF INTERVENTION FOR HYPERMOBILITY

First check for areas of hypomobility near the region of hypermobility. By improving the hypomobility, symptoms associated with the hypermobility may resolve.

When you are using physiologic or accessory motions, movement grades III to V should not be used with hypermobility because these grades move to the ends of the motion range and may increase the hypermobility.

When symptoms of increased tone or pain are present, movement grade I or II can be used to neuromodulate pain.[13]

Movement grades II and III – (staying short of the ends of range of motion) may improve the quality of the range of movement. The larger arc of movement provides proprioceptive sensation. Physiologic motion may be more advantageous than accessory motion because physiologic motion creates a greater arc of movement.

In addition to intervention by using joint mobilization, regional and local stabilization strengthening should be considered.[24] A corset or a brace may help to stabilize the region, as well as provide proprioceptive input.[25–28] Sclerosant injections may create fibrosis of collagen to modify joint mobility or chemically ablate nociception.[29–30] Surgery may be necessary to stabilize the joint.

RATIONALE FOR THE INTERVENTION EFFECTS OF MOBILIZATION AND MANIPULATION

Neurophysiologic Mechanisms for the Reduction of Pain and Muscle Spasm

Regarding acute pain, mobilization and manipulation activate sensory afferents from the skin, muscle, and joint receptors. Upon entering the spinal cord, there is interaction with other sensory inputs, which may result in summation or inhibition.[31] Mobilization and manipulation may cause activity in the inhibitory central systems that could include local spinal circuits[32] and/or activation of descending systems.[33-35]

Manipulation to the thoracic spine produces cellular biologic markers such as substance P and enhanced polymorphonuclear neutrophil respiratory burst.[36;37]

Research in chronic pain suggests that nociceptive activity is unlikely to be involved. Instead, chronic pain is a complex combination of biologic and psychosocial factors.[38;39] With chronic pain, the nervous system is sensitized.[38] Mobilization and manipulation may do little to alleviate pain in chronic states.

Biomechanical Considerations

Research (controlled randomized studies) has not shown that either mobilization or manipulation restores range of motion when hypomobility is present. From a biomechanical perspective, the use of movement grades III to V, movement at the end of range, is necessary to increase range of motion and has often been cited as a limitation to the current research.

Literature supports the beneficial effects of movement on healing. Passive motion stimulates tissue repair in skin,[40-42] tendons,[43-46] and ligaments,[47;48] and increased cellularity and cell products.[49] Continuous passive motion improves the rate and extent of healing of articular cartilage.[50;51] Improvements in ligament strength and linear stiffness of scars, matrix organization, and collagen concentration have been found with movement compared to immobilization techniques.[52] As mobilization and manipulation creates passive motion, these techniques may cause similar improvements. Further research is needed to determine the biomechanical effects of mobilization and manipulation.

Psychologic Considerations

The placebo effect has been estimated to create 20 to 30% of patient improvements during intervention.[53] The psychologic benefits associated with such factors as "the laying on of hands" and the charisma of the clinician all must be considered as part of the efficacy of mobilization and manipulation.[53;54]

RELIABILITY AND VALIDITY OF ACCESSORY MOTION INTERVENTION

There is a paucity of research available on interventions related to the spine. Results are limited because of problems with poor methodology, including the lack of control groups, randomization, blind outcome assessment, criteria for subject selection, description of the intervention, and statistical analysis and power.[55] The following studies represent the current knowledge regarding the spine and peripheral joints.

A meta-analysis for the cervical spine concluded that manipulation and mobilization probably provide at least short-term benefits for some patients with neck pain and headaches.[56] However, the studies may have been confounded by using a mixture of treatment types.[55] Manipulation was slightly more effective than mobilization or physical therapy for some patients with subacute or chronic neck pain (all three were superior to usual medical care).[56]

Data was combined from studies deemed to be similar in terms of types of patients with somatic pain syndromes to calculate pooled effect sizes. Treatment procedures produced a small to medium effect size to show that mobilization and manipulation are slightly better than control or comparison interventions. Mobilization and manipulation may also provide a short-term improvement in pain associated with head and neck disorders, but no difference was found between the two techniques.[55]

A meta-analysis for the lumbar spine concluded that manipulation has a short-term benefit in some patients, especially those with uncomplicated acute low-back pain (LBP) with no sciatic nerve irritation. But manipulation's long-term effect, either in preventing chronic LBP or in preventing recurrence of acute LBP, is unknown. The number of treatments required and whether they should end before or after the patient becomes pain free are unclear.[57]

A systematic review of randomized clinical trials with LBP indicated that manipulation was more effective than a range of reference treatments. No difference in effect could be determined when comparing manipulation with control treatment in a considerable number of trials. Most trials reported only short-term effects. Regarding acute LBP, evidence in favor of manipulation was inconclusive and there was insufficient evidence for patients with chronic LBP.[58]

A methodologic comparison among randomized and controlled studies on LBP interventions leading to return to work demonstrated meager scientific foundations on which industrial rehabilitation programs are based. The study review found (a) bedrest for a very brief period (1 to 3 days) is reasonable for non-neurologic LBP; (b) exercise as typically prescribed has a limited role in acute LBP; (c) there is no proven benefit of exercise for return to work after mild non-neurologic LBP; (d) a generalized aerobic and flexibility approach for long-term prevention of acute episodes of LBP appears to be warranted; (e) back school has not been proven to expedite return to work in acute LBP; and (f) data on the efficacy of back schools to reduce LBP recurrences are equivocal.[59]

A systematic review of randomized controlled trials for acute and chronic LBP concluded (a) that there was strong evidence for the effectiveness of muscle relaxants and nonsteroidal anti-inflammatory drugs, whereas exercise therapy for acute LBP was ineffective; and (b) there was strong evidence for the effectiveness of manipulation, back schools, and exercise therapy for chronic LBP, especially for short-term effects.[60] A meta-analysis concluded that a nonsurgical multidisciplinary team approach for chronic LBP more than doubled the number of patients who returned to work.[61]

A meta-analysis concluded that the effects in favor of mobilization and manipulation were greater (a) if other forms of treatment were provided in conjunction with the mobilization and manipulation and (b) when the treatment effects where measured immediately following therapy.[62]

The literature on peripheral joint mobilization is limited. Controlled trials on mobilization of the shoulder compared to a control group show no difference in shoulder function or active range of motion.[63–65] In treated subjects as compared to controls, mobilization improved the range of motion of the wrist and hand.[66]

Scientific evidence to support the efficacy of mobilization is nonexistent in pediatrics.[2]

INDICATIONS AND CONTRAINDICATIONS FOR JOINT MOBILIZATION

The indication and contraindication information for using accessory motion techniques included in the examination portion (see Chapter 1) are the same for intervention.

REFERENCES

1. Greenman PE: Principles of Manual Medicine. Baltimore, Williams & Wilkins, 1989.
2. Harris SR, Lundgren BD: Joint mobilization for children with central nervous system disorder: Indications and precautions. Physical Therapy 71(12):890–896, 1991.
3. Maitland GD: Vertebral Manipulation, 5th ed. London, Butterworths, 1986.
4. Condon SN, Hutton RS: Soleus muscle electromyographic activity and ankle dorsiflexion range of motion during four stretching procedures. Physical Therapy 67(1): 24–30, 1987.
5. Tannigawa M: Comparison of the hold-relax procedure and passive mobilization on increasing muscle length. Physical Therapy 52 (7):725–735, 1972.
6. Voss DE, Ionta MK, Myers BJ: Proprioceptive Neuromuscular Facilitation: Patterns and Techniques, 3rd ed. Philadelphia, Harper & Row, 1985.
7. Bandy WB, Irion JM: The effects of time on static stretch on the flexibility of the hamstring muscles. Physical Therapy 74:845–850, 1994.
8. Cherry D: Review of physical therapy alternatives for reducing muscle contracture. Physical Therapy 60 (7):877–881, 1980.

9. Kendall FP, McCreary EK, Provance PG: Muscles: Testing and Function with Posture and Pain, 4th ed. Baltimore, Williams & Willkins, 1993, pp. 33–37.
10. Hollenbery S, Dennis M: An introduction to craniosacral therapy. Physiotherapy 80(8):528–532, 1994.
11. Norkin CC, White DJ: Measurement of Joint Motion: A Guide to Goniometry. Philadelphia, FA Davis, 1985.
12. Warwick R, Williams PL, eds: Gray's Anatomy, 35th British Edition. Philadelphia, WB Saunders, 1995.
13. Melzack R, Wall PD: Pain mechanisms: A new theory: A gate control system modulates sensory input from the skin before it evokes pain perception and response. Science 150(3699):971–979, 1965.
14. Twomey L, Taylor J: Spine update: Exercise and spinal manipulation in the treatment of low back pain. Spine 29(5):615–619, 1995.
15. Gilbert MM, Scott RA: Analysis of the joint crack by simultaneous recording of sound and tension. Journal of Manipulative Physiological Therapy 9(3):189–195, 1986.
16. Sandoz R: The significance of the manipulative crack and of other articular noises. Annals of Swiss Chiropractic Association 4:47–68, 1969.
17. Petersen CM, Hayes KW: Construct validity of Cyriax's selective tension examination: Association of end-feels with pain at the knee and shoulder. Journal of Orthopaedic & Sports Physical Therapy 30(9):512–527, 2000.
18. Fritz JM, Delitto A, Erhard RE, et al: An examination of the selective tissue tension scheme, with evidence for the concept of a capsular pattern of the knee. Physical Therapy 79(10):1046–1061, 1998.
19. Hayes KW, Petersen CM, Falconer J: An examination of Cyriax's passive motion tests with patients having osteoarthritis of the knee. Physical Therapy 74(8):697–709, 1994.
20. Maitland GD: The importance of adding compression when examining and treating synovial joints. In: Glasgow EF (ed): Aspects of Manipulative Therapy 2nd ed. Melbourne, Churchill Livingstone, 1985, pp. 109–115.
21. MacConaill MA, Basmajian JV: Muscles and Movement: A Basis for Human Kinesiology. Baltimore, Williams & Wilkins, 1969.
22. Evans P: Ligaments, joint surfaces, conjunct rotation and close-pack. Physiotherapy 74(3):105–114, 1988.
23. Paris SV: Mobilization of the spine. Physical Therapy 59(8):988–995, 1979.
24. O'Sullivan PB, Twomey LT, Allison GT: Evaluation of specific stabilizing exercise in the treatment of chronic low back pain with radiologic diagnosis of spondylolysis or spondylolisthesis. Spine 22(24):2959–2967, 1997.
25. McNair PJ, Heine PJ: Trunk proprioception: Enhancement through lumbar bracing. Archives of Physical Medicine & Rehabilitation 80:96–99, 1999.
26. Jerosch J, Prymka M: Knee proprioception in normal volunteers and patients with anterior cruciate ligament tears, taking special account of the effect of a knee bandage. Archives of Orthopedic Trauma Surgery 115:162–166, 1996.
27. Perlau R, Frank C, Fick G: The effect of elastic bandages on human knee proprioception in the uninjured population. American Orthopaedic Society for Sports Medicine 23(2):251–255, 1995.
28. Lephart SM, Pincivero DM, Giraldo JL, et al: The role of proprioception in the management and rehabilitation of athletic injuries. The American Journal of Sports Medicine 25:130–137, 1997.

29. Barbor R: Low backache. British Medical Journal i:55, 1955.
30. Barbor R: Treatment for chronic low back pain. Paris, Proceedings of IVth International Congress of Physical Medicine, 1964.
31. Wall PD: Overview of pain and its mechanisms. In: Shacklock MO, ed: Moving in on Pain. Chatswood, Australia, Butterworth-Heinemann, 1995, p. 13.
32. Watkins LR, Mayer DJ: Organisation of endogenous opiate and nonopiate pain control systems. Science 216:1185–1192, 1982.
33. Fields HL, Basbaum AI: Central nervous system mechanisms of pain modulation, in Wall PD, Melzack R, eds: Textbook of Pain. Edinburgh, Churchill Livingstone, 1994.
34. Wall PD: Treatment of pain, in Shacklock MO, ed: Moving in on Pain. Chatswood, Australia, Butterworth-Heinemann, 1995, p. 64.
35. Wright A: Hypoalgesia post-manipulative therapy: A review of potential neurophysiological mechanisms. Manual Therapy 1:11–16, 1995.
36. Brennan PC, Kokjohn K, Kaltinger CJ, et al.: Enhanced phagocytic cell respiratory burst induced by spinal manipulation: Potential role of substance P. Journal of Manipulative Physiological Therapy 14(7):399–408, 1991.
37. Brennan PC, Triano JJ, McGregor M, et al: Enhanced neutrophil respiratory burst as a biological marker for manipulation forces: Duration of the effect and association with substance P and tumor necrosis factor. Journal of Manipulative and Physiological Therapeutics 15(2):83–89, 1992.
38. Gifford L: Pain, the tissues and the nervous system: A conceptual model. Physiotherapy 84(1):27–36, 1998.
39. Zusman M: Instigators of activity intolerance. Manual Therapy 2(2):75–86, 1997.
40. Arem AJ, Madden JW: Effects of stress on healing wounds: I. Intermittent noncyclical tension. Journal of Surgical Research 20:93, 1976.
41. Forrester JC, Szederfeldt BH, Hayes TL, et al: Wolff's law in relation to the healing skin wound. Journal of Trauma 10:770, 1970.
42. Lagrana NA, Alexander H, Strauchler I, et al: Effect of mechanical load in wound healing. Annals of Plastic Surgery 10:200, 1983.
43. Gelberman RH, Amiel D, Gonsalves M, et al: The influence of protected passive mobilization on the healing of flexor tendons. A biochemical and microangiographic study. Hand 13:120, 1981.
44. Gelberman RH, Woo SL-Y, Lothringer K, et al.: Effects of early intermittent passive mobilization on healing canine flexor tendons. Journal of Hand Surgery 7:170, 1982.
45. Kessler I, Missim F: Primary repair without immobilization of flexor tendon division within the digital sheath. Acta Orthopedica Scandanavia 40:587, 1969.
46. Stickland JW, Glogovac SV: Digital function following flexor tendon repair in zone 2: A comparison of immobilization and controlled passive motion techniques. Journal of Hand Surgery 5:537, 1980.
47. Fronek J, Frank C, Amiel D, et al: The effect of intermittent passive motion (IPM) in the healing of the medial collateral ligament [abstract]. Proceedings of Orthopedic Research Society 8:31, 1983.
48. Mueller ME, Allgower M, Willeneggar H: Manual of Internal Fixation. New York, Springer-Verlag, 1970, p. 2.
49. Frank C, Akeson WH, Woo SL-Y, et al: Physiology and therapeutic value of passive joint motion. Clinical Orthopedics 185:113–125, 1984.
50. Salter RB: The biological effects of continuous passive motion. Journal of Bone & Joint Surgery A 62:1232–1251, 1980.

51. Salter RB, Simmonds DF, Malcolm BW, et al: The biological effects of continuous passive motion in the healing of full thickness defects in articular cartilage. Journal of Bone & Joint Surgery A 62:1232, 1980.

52. Long ML, Frank C, Schachar NS, et al.: The effect of motion on normal and healing ligaments. Proceedings of Orthopedic Research Society 7:43, 1982.

53. Wells PE: Manipulative procedures, In Wells PE, Frampton V, Bowsher D, eds: Pain Management in Physical Therapy. E. Norwalk, CT, Appleton & Lange, 1988, pp. 181–217.

54. Zusman M: Spinal manipulative therapy: Review of some proposed mechanisms and a new hypothesis. Australian Journal of Physiotherapy 32:89–99, 1986.

55. Di Fabio RD: Efficacy of manual therapy. Physical Therapy 72(12):853–860, 1992.

56. Hurwitz EJ, Aker SD, Adams AH, et al.: Manipulation and mobilization of the cervical spine: A systematic review of the literature. Spine 21(15):1746–1760, 1996.

57. Shekelle PG, Adams AH, Chassin MR, et al: Spinal manipulation for low-back pain. Annals of Internal Medicine 117(7):590–598, 1992.

58. Koes BW, Assendelft WJJ, van der Heijden GJMG, et al: Spinal manipulation for low back pain: An updated systematic review of randomized clinical trials. Spine 21(24): 2860–2873, 1996.

59. Scheer SJ, Radack KL, O'Brien DR: Randomized controlled trials in industrial low back pain relating to return to work. Part 1. Acute interventions. Archives of Physical Medicine & Rehabilitation 76:966–973, 1995.

60. van Tulder MW, Koes BW, Bouter LM: Conservative treatment of acute and chronic nonspecific low back pain: A systematic review of randomized controlled trials of the most common interventions. Spine 22(18):2128–2156, 1997.

61. Cutler RB, Fishbain DA, Rosomoff HL, et al: Does nonsurgical pain center treatment of chronic pain return patients to work: A review and meta-analysis of the literature. Spine 19(6):643–652, 1993.

62. Ottenbacher K, DiFabio RP: Efficacy of spinal manipulation/mobilization therapy: A meta-analysis. Spine 19(9):833–837, 1985.

63. Bulgen DY, Binder AI, Hazleman BL, et al: Frozen shoulder: Prospective clinical study with an evaluation of three treatment regimens. Annals of Rheumatology Disease 43:353–360, 1984.

64. Conroy DE, Hayes KW: The effect of joint mobilization as a component of comprehensive treatment for primary shoulder impingement syndrome. Journal of Orthopaedic & Sports Physical Therapy 28:3–13, 1998.

65. Nicholson GG: The effects of passive joint mobilization on pain and hypomobility associated with adhesive capsulitis of the shoulder. Journal of Orthopaedic & Sports Physical Therapy 6:238–246, 1985.

66. Randall T, Portney L, Harris BA: Effects of joint mobilization on joint stiffness and active motion of the metacarpal-phalangeal joint. Journal of Orthopaedic & Sports Physical Therapy 16:30–36, 1982.

NEURODYNAMIC PRINCIPLES OF MOBILIZATION FOR INTERVENTION

APPROACHES TO MOBILIZATION OF THE NERVOUS SYSTEM

Principles of movement that apply to joints, tendons, or muscles apply to the movement of nerves. The neural elements must accommodate to changes in the length of the nerve bed with body movement. The brachial plexus has an average excursion of 15 mm when the upper extremity is moved from full abduction to full adduction.[1] When treating injuries involving the nerve or the nerve bed, concepts of nervous system mobilization must be considered.[2;3] The goal of treatment is to restore normal elasticity, range of motion, and communication within the nervous system. An overall approach is to return the nervous system from a state of pathodynamics to a state of normal neurodynamics.

Neural mobilization techniques are considered intervention when the examination information supports a hypothesis of pathodynamics in the clinical reasoning/problem solving format.[4] Neurodynamic techniques are just one part of a comprehensive intervention program. Components of education, posture correction, ergonomics, and a home program, for example, are all vitally important for a successful outcome.

TYPES OF ACTIVATING FORCES

There are two ways to use movement in the treatment of positive neural disorders. One way is direct mobilization of the nerve through the use of neurodynamic examination techniques. The other, an indirect approach, addresses the neural interface, tissues that surround or "interface" with the nerve such as the nerve bed, joints, muscles, fascia, subcutaneous tissue, fibro-osseous tunnels, and skin.[5] Clinicians should identify tissues along a nerve's tract that are possible areas of pathology affecting nerve function, or that create problems of pathomechanics or pathophysiology. Additionally, mobilization occurs with other approaches, such as active or passive mobilization of the various joint complexes, massage, muscle stretching, or posture reeducation.

An overall intervention approach uses both direct and indirect nerve mobilization to insure the best possible outcome.

CONSIDERATIONS FOR NEURAL MOBILIZATION

The principles regarding joint mobilization (see Chapters 1 and 4) apply to mobilization of the nervous system. Combinations of active, passive, and muscle-energy techniques can be used as well. Neural mobilization techniques should be gentle, especially during the first several sessions. The clinician must monitor all signs and symptoms. The concepts of severity, irritability, and nature should be considered.[6]

Clinicians should be aware of variations in the end-feel categories;[7] for example, the difference in the sensation experienced with an abnormal early capsular versus a muscle spasm end-feel. End-feel responses felt when the nervous system is loaded may present as new and subtle sensations.

Intervention should be completed without symptom reproduction. Techniques will include movements in various parts of the range, including end-range mobilization. If intervention starts to provoke symptoms, modification of the amplitude, range, or speed of the movement must be altered to a level of non-symptom reproduction. The principle that neural tissue is mobilized, not stretched, must always be followed.

For an acute injury, start the technique away from the local area of involvement or pathology. An acute to subacute ankle sprain may require a straight leg raise technique that takes up the slack in the lumbar spine, the hip, and the knee. The ankle position should be maintained in neutral or plantar flexion. As the condition becomes more chronic in nature, slack may be able to be taken up first in the ankle, and followed, in order, by the knee and the hip. Use the connective tissue continuum of the nervous system as a mechanical link to the involved areas of adverse pathomechanics.

The clinical presentation of an acute, irritable disorder (considered a pathophysiological dominated state) should be treated with gentle movements. This helps to decrease any pain-producing impulse that can be activated by a sensitive nervous system. On the contrary, a chronic nonirritable disorder (considered a pathomechanical-dominated state) may tolerate greater tension with end-range loaded movements, including grade IV movements.[6]

Initially with an acute presentation, the clinician should start to slide the neural elements through ranges of movement using grades II and III.[6] The focus is to provide elongation, longitudinal excursion, and movement, but not to tension the nervous tissue.[8] This is important for maintaining blood flow and nutrition to the neural elements as well as axoplasmic flow. Intervention must address both pathomechanics and pathophysiology.

Initially, techniques are performed passively. Progression to active techniques and functional movements should be incorporated as quickly as appropriate. Home programs with self-mobilization of the nervous system should be started early in the intervention, as should patient education.

Patient motivation is critical. Ultimately, the patient must be responsible for the success and/or failure of the intervention program. Patient compliance with therapy is necessary to insure a successful outcome. Patients must understand their problem and assume control of their own care.[9;10]

PROGRESSION OF INTERVENTION

There are a variety of ways to address intervention progression including the number of repetitions, amplitude of movement, tissue tension, and time of technique performance.

Initially, the number of repetitions may be as few as 1 to 5, but should be increased quickly to 10 to 20. This also relates to the number of sets of repetitions or the number of times performed per day. The overall amplitude should be increased through a greater excursion of the range.

An increase in resistance relating to an increase in tension to the nerve can be progressed by changing the joint's position through the neural continuum. For example, adding medial rotation of the hip to a straight leg raise increases the load on the neural elements.

From an endurance perspective, the repetitions can be based on time that may last up to several minutes, a pacing program that does not focus on pain as a guide. Endurance affects the metabolic factor of a nerve.

The number of repetitions or sets of repetitions should be determined by the health of the nervous system. Provocation or symptom generation is an expression of the amount of pathophysiology and relates to components of nerve ischemosensitivity, mechanosensitivity, or chemosensitivity. Continual reassessment is necessary to provide appropriate intervention. The pathophysiology of the nerve and the nerve's expression of dysfunction provide the clinician with criteria to change the examination or intervention process[10;11] and to determine the optimal number of repetitions, sets, or time factor for intervention.

NERVOUS SYSTEM MOBILIZATION RESEARCH

The following studies are examples of the current research on intervention using mobilization of the nervous system.

A study analyzing outcomes for hamstring injuries used traditional treatment versus traditional treatment with the addition of neural mobilization. The results found slump-stretching techniques combined with traditional intervention superior to traditional intervention alone.[12] To the contrary, another study found no difference in outcomes between an experimental group using neural mobilization and a control group of patients, 6 weeks postspinal surgery.[13]

A study involving neural mobilization of the ulnar nerve with medial elbow pain found a correlation between positive preoperative findings and postoperative findings. The ulnar nerve was found to be entrapped at the elbow at the time of surgery and following surgical release, the upper limb neurodynamic test for the ulnar nerve responded normally to loading.

The body of research regarding neural mobilization is expanding but ongoing research is essential to validate this new intervention.

INDICATIONS AND CONTRAINDICATIONS FOR MOBILIZATION OF THE NERVOUS SYSTEM

The indication and contraindication information for using mobilization in the nervous system, included in the neurodynamics examination portion (see Chapter 2), are the same for intervention.

REFERENCES

1. Wilgis E, Murphy R: The significance of longitudinal excursion in peripheral nerves. Hand Clinics 2:761–786, 1986.
2. Wilgis EFS: Clinical aspects of nerve gliding in the upper extremity. In: Hunter J, Schneider L, Mackin E, eds: Tendon and Nerve Surgery in the Hand. St. Louis, Mosby, 1997, pp. 121–124.
3. Byron P: Upper extremity nerve gliding. In: Hunter J, Schneider L, Mackin, E, eds: Tendon and Nerve Surgery in the Hand. St. Louis, Mosby, 1997, pp. 125–133.
4. Jones M: Clinical reasoning in manual therapy. Physical Therapy 72:875–884, 1992.
5. Butler DS: Mobilisation of the Nervous System. Melbourne, Australia, Churchill Livingstone, 1991.
6. Maitland GD: Vertebral Manipulation, 5th ed. London, Butterworths, 1986.
7. Cyriax J: Textbook of Orthopaedic Medicine, 8th ed. London, Baillière Tindall, 1982.
8. Lundborg G: Nerve Injury and Repair. New York, Churchill Livingstone, 1988.
9. Campbell J: Pain 1996 — An Updated Review: Refresher Course Syllabus. Seattle, IASP Press, 1996.
10. Foley R: Complex Regional Pain Syndromes: Focus on the Autonomic Nervous System. Adelaide, Australia, NOI Group Publications, 2000.
11. Butler DS: The Sensitive Nervous System. Adelaide, Australia, NOI Group Publications, 2000.
12. Kornberg C, Lew P: The effect of stretching neural structures on grade one hamstring injuries. Journal of Orthopaedic and Sports Physical Therapy 10:481–487, 1989.
13. Maher C, Scrimshaw S: Does neural mobilization influence the outcome of spinal surgery. 13th World Conference of Physical Therapy, Yokahama, Japan, 1999.
14. Shacklock M: Positive upper limb tension test in a case of surgically proven neuropathy. Manual Therapy 1:154–161, 1996.

A P P E N D I X 1

NORMAL END-FEELS ASSOCIATED WITH PHYSIOLOGIC MOTIONS

END-FEEL (CYRIAX)	PHYSIOLOGIC MOTION (EXCLUDING MULTIJOINT MUSCLE IMPLICATIONS)
	METACARPALS/INTERPHALANGEALS/ CARPOMETACARPALS
Hard capsular	Flexion
Capsular	Extension
Capsular	Abduction
Capsular	Adduction
	RADIOCARPAL/MIDCARPAL
Capsular	Flexion
Hard capsular	Extension
Capsular	Ulnar Deviation
Hard capsular	Radial Deviation
	ELBOW
Tissue approximation	Flexion
Bone-to-bone	Extension
Hard capsular	Pronation
Capsular	Supination
	SHOULDER
Capsular	Flexion
Capsular	Extension
Capsular	Abduction
Hard capsular/Tissue approximation	Horizontal Adduction
Capsular	External Rotation
Capsular	Internal Rotation
	METATARSOPHALANGEAL/ INTERPHALANGEAL
Hard capsular	Flexion
Capsular	Extension
Capsular	Abduction
Capsular	Adduction

END-FEEL (CYRIAX)	PHYSIOLOGIC MOTION (EXCLUDING MULTIJOINT MUSCLE IMPLICATIONS)
	ANKLE
Capsular/Muscular	Dorsiflexion
Capsular	Plantar Flexion
Capsular	Eversion
Capsular	Inversion
	KNEE
Tissue approximation	Flexion
Springy capsular	Extension
Capsular	External Rotation
Capsular	Internal Rotation
	HIP
Tissue approximation/Capsular	Flexion
Capsular	Extension
Capsular	Abduction
Capsular	Adduction
Capsular	External Rotation
Hard capsular	Internal Rotation
	SPINE
Capsular	Flexion
Bone-to-bone	Extension
Capsular/Muscular (cervical)	Side Bending
Capsular	Rotation
	TEMPOROMANDIBULAR
Capsular	Opening
Capsular	Protrusion
Hard capsular	Retrusion

JOINT CLOSE- AND LOOSE-PACKED POSITIONS

JOINT POSITION	CLOSE-PACKED	LOOSE-PACKED
UPPER EXTREMITY		
Interphalangeal I–V	Full extension	Slight flexion
Metacarpophalangeal I	Full extension	Slight flexion
Metacarpophalangeal II–V	Full flexion	Slight flexion and slight ulnar deviation
Carpometacarpal I	Full opposition	Neutral
Radiocarpal	Full extension and radial deviation	Slight flexion and slight ulnar deviation
Midcarpal	Full extension	Slight flexion
Distal Radioulnar	0–5° supination	10–35° supination
Humeroulnar	Full extension and full supination	70° flexion and 10–35° supination
Humeroradial	90° flexion and 0–5° supination	Full extension and full supination
Proximal Radioulnar	0–5° supination	70° flexion and 10–35° supination
Glenohumeral	Full abduction and full external rotation	55° abduction and 30° horizontal adduction
Subacromial	90° abduction	Anatomic position
Acromioclavicular	90° abduction	Anatomic position
Sternoclavicular	Full elevation	Anatomic position
Scapulothoracic	Full elevation	Anatomic position
LOWER EXTREMITY		
Interphalangeal I–V	Full extension	Slight flexion
Metatarsophalangeal I–V	Full extension	Slight extension (10°)
Midtarsal	Supination of the subtalar joint	Pronation of the subtalar joint or a mid-range position of the ankle/foot
Tarsometatarsal	Plantar flexion	Dorsiflexion
Subtalar	Full supination	Midway between supination and pronation
Talocrural	Full dorsiflexion	10° plantar flexion and midway between supination and pronation

JOINT POSITION	CLOSE-PACKED	LOOSE-PACKED
Distal Tibiofibular	Full dorsiflexion	10° plantar flexion
Proximal Tibiofibular	Full dorsiflexion	Knee midway between flexion and extension and 10° plantar flexion
Femoral/Tibial	Full extension and slight tibial external rotation	20–30° flexion
Patella/Femoral	90°flexion	Full extension and full tibial external rotation
Hip	Full extension, slight internal rotation, and slight abduction	30°flexion, 30° abduction, and slight external rotation
SPINE	Extension	Neutral to slight flexion
TEMPOROMANDIBULAR	Retrusion with full occlusion	Nearly centric occlusion

PHYSIOLOGIC AND ACCESSORY MOTION CORRELATIONS

The following physiologic and accessory motion correlations for the extremity joints are made related to the most common anatomic/kinesiologic findings at each joint complex.

Only indications for hypomobility are included, but hypermobility may also be associated with any of the techniques.

Physiologic and accessory motions may not correlate in the spine because of the three-joint complex interaction of the two zygapophyseal joints and the intervertebral disc.

ACCESSORY TECHNIQUE	INDICATION(S)
METACARPALPHALANGEAL I-V/INTERPHALANGEAL I-V	
Distraction	Any capsular hypomobility
Compression	Provocation findings with arthritis
Dorsal Glide	Extension hypomobility
Volar Glide	Flexion hypomobility
Ulnar Glide	Thumb flexion hypomobility, II and III ulnar deviation (adduction) hypomobility, and IV and V ulnar deviation (abduction) hypomobility
Radial Glide	Thumb extension hypomobility, II and III radial deviation (abduction) hypomobility, and IV and V radial deviation (adduction) hypomobility
Medial Rotation	Thumb flexion hypomobility and II to V extension hypomobility
Lateral Rotation	Thumb extension hypomobility and II to V flexion hypomobility
CARPOMETACARPAL I	
Distraction	Any capsular hypomobility
Compression	Provocation findings with arthritis
Dorsal Glide	Thumb abduction hypomobility
Palmar/Volar Glide	Thumb adduction hypomobility
Ulnar Glide	Thumb flexion hypomobility

ACCESSORY TECHNIQUE	INDICATION(S)
Radial Glide	Thumb extension hypomobility
Medial Rotation	Thumb flexion hypomobility
Lateral Rotation	Thumb extension hypomobility
INTERMETACARPAL I-V	
Dorsal Glide	I to V extension hypomobility
Volar Glide	I to V flexion hypomobility
RADIOCARPAL (RC)/MIDCARPAL (MC)	
Distraction	Any capsular hypomobility
Compression	Provocation findings with arthritis
Dorsal Glide	Wrist (especially the RC joint and the medial portion of the MC joint) flexion hypomobility
Palmar/Volar Glide	Wrist (especially the RC joint and the medial portion of MC joint) extension hypomobility
Ulnar Glide	RC radial deviation hypomobility and MC ulnar deviation hypomobility
Radial Glide	RC ulnar deviation hypomobility and MC radial deviation hypomobility
Supination	Supination hypomobility
Pronation	Pronation hypomobility
DISTAL RADIOULNAR	
Compression	Provocation findings with arthritis
Dorsal Glide	Supination hypomobility
Palmar/Volar Glide	Pronation hypomobility
HUMEROULNAR	
Distraction	Any capsular hypomobility
Compression	Provocation findings with arthritis
Cephalic Glide	Extension end-range hypomobility, flexion end-range hypomobility, and supination hypomobility
Caudal Glide	Extension beginning range hypomobility, flexion beginning range hypomobility, and pronation hypomobility
Medial Tilt/Valgus Stress Test	Extension hypomobility and supination hypomobility; medial collateral ligament involvement with stress testing
Lateral Tilt/Varus Stress Test	Flexion hypomobility and pronation hypomobility; lateral collateral ligament involvement with stress testing

ACCESSORY TECHNIQUE	INDICATION(S)
HUMERORADIAL	
Distraction	Any capsular hypomobility
Compression	Provocation findings with arthritis
Dorsal Glide	Extension hypomobility
Palmar/Volar Glide	Flexion hypomobility
Rotation	Pronation hypomobility or supination hypomobility
Lateral Tilt/Varus Stress Test	Lateral collateral ligament stress testing
PROXIMAL RADIOULNAR	
Dorsal Glide	Pronation hypomobility
Volar Glide	Supination hypomobility
Cephalic Glide	Pronation hypomobility
Caudal Glide	Supination hypomobility
Rotation	Pronation hypomobility or supination hypomobility
GLENOHUMERAL	
Lateral Distraction	Any capsular hypomobility
Compression	Provocation finding with arthritis
Anterior Glide	Flexion end range hypomobility, extension hypomobility, external rotation hypomobility, and horizontal abduction hypomobility
Posterior Glide	Flexion hypomobility, internal rotation hypomobility, and horizontal adduction hypomobility
Inferior Glide	Abduction hypomobility, flexion hypomobility, and extension hypomobility
SUBACROMIAL	
Long Axis Distraction	Subacromial impingement and inferior glenohumeral capsular hypomobility
Long Axis Compression	Provocation findings with subacromial impingement
ACROMIOCLAVICULAR	
Distraction/Anterior Glide	Any capsular hypomobility (distraction); protraction hypomobility (anterior glide)
Compression/Posterior Glide	Provocation findings with arthritis (compression); retraction hypomobility (posterior glide)
Cephalic/Caudal Glide	Elevation hypomobility (cephalic); depression hypomobility (caudal)

ACCESSORY TECHNIQUE	INDICATION(S)
STERNOCLAVICULAR	
Distraction	Any capsular hypomobility
Compression	Provocation findings with arthritis
Anterior Glide	Protraction hypomobility
Posterior Glide	Retraction hypomobility
Superior Glide	Depression hypomobility
Inferior Glide	Elevation hypomobility
SCAPULOTHORACIC	
Distraction	Any capsular hypomobility
Superior Glide	Hypomobility in any scapular depression muscles
Inferior Glide	Hypomobility in any scapular elevator muscles
Medial Glide	Hypomobility in any scapular protractor muscles
Lateral Glide	Hypomobility in any scapular retractor muscles
Medial Rotation	Hypomobility in any scapular lateral rotator muscles
Lateral Rotation	Hypomobility in any scapular medial rotator muscles
HIP	
Long Axis Traction	To decrease superior femoral contact surface area and inferior capsular hypomobility
Long Axis Compression	Provocation findings with superior femoral contact area changes
Lateral Distraction	Any capsular hypomobility
Compression	Provocation findings with arthritis
Anterior Glide	Extension hypomobility and external rotation hypomobility
Posterior Glide	Flexion hypomobility and internal rotation hypomobility
External Rotation	External rotation hypomobility
Internal Rotation	Internal rotation hypomobility
FEMORAL/TIBIAL	
Distraction	Any capsular hypomobility
Compression	Provocation findings with arthritis
Anterior Glide	Extension hypomobility
Posterior Glide	Flexion hypomobility
Medial/Lateral Rotation	Flexion hypomobility (medial); extension hypomobility (lateral)
Medial Tilt/Valgus Stress Test	Extension hypomobility; medial capsule and collateral ligament involvement with stress testing

ACCESSORY TECHNIQUE	INDICATION(S)
Lateral Tilt/Varus Stress Test	Flexion hypomobility; lateral capsule and collateral ligament involvement with stress testing
PATELLA/FEMORAL	
Distraction	Any capsular hypomobility
Compression	Provocation findings of arthritis
Cephalic Glide	Extension hypomobility
Caudal Glide	Flexion hypomobility
Medial Glide	Extension hypomobility and flexion hypomobility
Lateral Glide/Apprehension Test	Extension hypomobility and flexion hypomobility; provocation findings with subluxation/dislocation hypermobility
PROXIMAL TIBIOFIBULAR	
Anterior Glide	Plantar flexion hypomobility
Posterior Glide	Dorsiflexion hypomobility
Cephalic Glide	Dorsiflexion hypomobility and eversion hypomobility
Caudal Glide	Plantar flexion hypomobility and inversion hypomobility
DISTAL TIBIOFIBULAR	
Compression	Provocation findings with arthritis and syndesmosis rupture
Anterior Glide	Dorsiflexion hypomobility
Posterior Glide	Plantar flexion hypomobility
TALOCRURAL	
Distraction	Any capsular hypomobility
Compression	Provocation findings with arthritis
Anterior Glide/Anterior Drawer Stress Test	Plantar flexion hypomobility; lateral collateral ligament involvement with stress testing
Posterior Glide	Dorsiflexion hypomobility
SUBTALAR	
Distraction	Any capsular hypomobility
Compression	Provocation findings with arthritis
Medial Glide	Eversion hypomobility
Lateral Glide	Inversion hypomobility
NAVICULAR/TALUS	
Dorsal Glide	Pronation hypomobility
Plantar Glide	Supination hypomobility
CUNEIFORMS/NAVICULAR	
Dorsal Glide	Pronation hypomobility
Plantar Glide	Supination hypomobility

ACCESSORY TECHNIQUE	INDICATION(S)
CUBOID/NAVICULAR-CUNEIFORM III	
Dorsal Glide	Pronation hypomobility
Plantar Glide	Supination hypomobility
METATARSAL I-III/CUNEIFORM I-III	
Dorsal Glide	Pronation hypomobility
Plantar Glide	Supination hypomobility
METATARSAL IV-V/CUBOID	
Dorsal Glide	Pronation hypomobility
Plantar Glide	Supination hypomobility
CUBOID/CALCANEUS	
Dorsal Glide	Supination hypomobility
Plantar Glide	Pronation hypomobility
INTERMETATARSAL I-V	
Dorsal/Plantar Glides	Pronation hypomobility (dorsal); supination hypomobility (plantar)
METATARSOPHALANGEAL I-V/INTERPHALANGEAL I-V	
Distraction	Any capsular hypomobility
Compression	Provocation findings with arthritis
Dorsal Glide	Extension hypomobility
Plantar Glide	Flexion hypomobility
Medial Glide	I and II abduction hypomobility and III to V adduction hypomobility
Lateral Glide	I and II adduction hypomobility and III to V abduction hypomobility
Medial Rotation	Extension hypomobility
Lateral Rotation	Flexion hypomobility
TEMPOROMANDIBULAR	
Distraction	Any capsular hypomobility
Compression	Provocation findings with arthritis
Anterior Glide	Protrusion hypomobility and opening hypomobility
Posterior Glide	Retrusion hypomobility
Medial Glide	Medial glide hypomobility
Lateral Glide	Lateral glide hypomobility

CAPSULAR PATTERNS

JOINT	PATTERN Pain may be present with any of the movement patterns
RIGHT TEMPOROMANDIBULAR	Deflection to the right with opening, deflection to the right with protrusion, and limited side glide to the left
CERVICAL	
Bilateral Zygapophyseal Involvement	Lateral flexions and rotations are equally limited, extension is limited, and flexion is usually full range but painful
Right Unilateral Zygapophyseal Involvement	Right lateral flexion, right rotation, and extension limited

THORACIC AND LUMBAR
Because of the effects of the degenerative process (aging) and habitual posturing, it is often difficult to determine whether range of motion is limited in these areas. A noncapsular pattern of limitation is easier to detect (see below Noncapsular Pattern: Thoracic and Lumbar).

Bilateral Zygapophyseal Involvement	Lateral flexions and rotations are equally limited, extension limited, and flexion is usually full range but painful
Right Unilateral Zygapophyseal Involvement	Right lateral flexion, left rotation, and extension limited
Sternoclavicular (SC)/Acromioclavicular (AC)	Pain at the extremes of elevation (SC/AC) and horizontal adduction (AC)
Glenohumeral	Lateral rotation >abduction/flexion >internal rotation limitations
Humeroulnar/Humeroradial	More limitation of flexion than of extension, and in the early stages of arthritis, rotation remains full and painless
Distal Radioulnar	A full range of motion with pain at both extremes of rotation
Radiocarpal/Midcarpal	An equal degree of limitation of flexion and extension

| | **PATTERN** |
JOINT	Pain may be present with any of the movement patterns
Carpometacarpal I	Limitation of abduction and extension with full flexion
Thumb and Finger Metacarpophalangeal/ Interphalangeal	More limitation of flexion than of extension
Sacroiliac/Symphysis Pubis/ Saccroccygeal	Pain when the joint is stressed
Hip	Gross limitation of flexion, abduction, and internal rotation; slight limitation of extension; little or no limitation of external rotation
Tibiofemoral	Gross limitation of flexion and slight limitation of extension; and in the early stages of arthritis, rotation remains full and painless
Tibiofibular	Pain occurs when contraction of the biceps femoris stretches the superior tibiofibular ligament; and pain occurs when the mortice is sprung at the talocrural joint stretching the inferior tibiofibular ligament
Talocrural	If the gastrocnemius muscle is of adequate length, there is more limitation of plantar flexion than of dorsiflexion
Subtalar	Limitation of supination (varus) increasing until in gross arthritis, the joint fixes in full pronation (valgus)
Midtarsal	Limitation of dorsiflexion, plantar flexion, adduction, and inversion; abduction and eversion are full range
Metatarsophalangeal I	Marked limitation of extension and slight limitation of flexion
Metatarsophalangeal II-V	Tend to fix in extension
Interphalangeal II-V	Tendency to flex

NONCAPSULAR PATTERN
The cause of this pattern is internal derangement, a disc protrusion or herniation.

Thoracic and Lumbar	Gross limitation of lateral flexion in one direction with full range in the other direction; or full extension range accompanied by markedly limited flexion. In the thoracic spine, rotation is limited in one direction.

INDEX